MX 0725566

D1615016

PRACTICE OSCEs IN
obstetrics and gynaecology

PRACTICE OSCEs IN
obstetrics and gynaecology

A guide for the medical student and MRANZCOG exams

Gareth Weston

Beverley Vollenhoven

Jane McNeilage

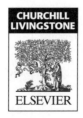

Sydney Edinburgh London New York Philadelphia St Louis Toronto

Churchill Livingstone
is an imprint of Elsevier

Elsevier Australia. ACN 001 002 357
(a division of Reed International Books Australia Pty Ltd)
Tower 1, 475 Victoria Avenue, Chatswood, NSW 2067

ELSEVIER

© 2009 Elsevier Australia

This publication is copyright. Except as expressly provided in the Copyright Act 1968
and the Copyright Amendment (Digital Agenda) Act 2000, no part of this publication
may be reproduced, stored in any retrieval system or transmitted by any means (including
electronic, mechanical, microcopying, photocopying, recording or otherwise) without prior
written permission from the publisher.

Every attempt has been made to trace and acknowledge copyright, but in some cases this
may not have been possible. The publisher apologises for any accidental infringement
and would welcome any information to redress the situation.

This publication has been carefully reviewed and checked to ensure that the content is as
accurate and current as possible at time of publication. We would recommend, however,
that the reader verify any procedures, treatments, drug dosages or legal content described
in this book. Neither the author, the contributors, nor the publisher assume any liability
for injury and/or damage to persons or property arising from any error in or omission
from this publication.

National Library of Australia Cataloguing-in-Publication Data

Weston, Gareth.

Practice OSCEs in obstetrics and gynaecology : a guide for
the medical student and MRANZCOG exams / Gareth Weston,
Beverley Vollenhoven, Jane McNeilage.

ISBN: 978 0 7295 3867 1 (pbk.)

Practice OSCEs Series.

Includes index.
Bibliography.

Royal Australian and New Zealand College of Obstetricians
and Gynaecologists--Examinations, questions, etc.
Obstetrics--Examinations, questions, etc.
Gynaecology--Examinations, questions, etc.

Vollenhoven, Beverley.
McNeilage, Jane.

618.076

Publisher: Sophie Kaliniecki
Developmental Editor: Sunalie Silva
Publishing Services Manager: Helena Klijn
Editorial Coordinator: Lauren Allsop
Edited by Margaret Trudgeon
Proofread by Sarah Newton-John
Internal and cover designs by Toni Darben
Index by Forsyth Publishing Services
Typeset by TnQ Books and Journals Pvt Ltd
Printed in Australia by Ligare

Site WH	MIDDLESEX UNIVERSITY LIBRARY
Accession No.	07255667
Class No.	WQ 18·Z WES
Special Collection ✓	

Contents

Foreword

Perhaps the only constant in the many recent changes in medical undergraduate and postgraduate education is the continuing demand for assessment. Undergraduate curricula in obstetrics and gynecology, now often broadened into Women's Health, typically only occupy 8 to 10 weeks in a four- or five-year medical course. Compressing principles and basic knowledge into this time is challenging for all universities. It has led some to develop National Collaborative Core Curricula to emphasise wellness and maintenance of health, while allowing for regional differences in health care needs (www.whccc.org/toc.cfm). Despite such learning challenges, all universities and colleges increasingly demand assessment that can withstand scrutiny.

Objective Structured Clinical Examinations (OSCEs) have become widely used since their introduction as an assessment tool about 30 years ago. Dr Gareth Weston and his colleagues are among the first generation of doctors who have grown up with OSCEs as medical students, and then as postgraduates, and now as examiners themselves in Obstetrics and Gynecology. They are ideally placed to write this invaluable resource in Obstetrics and Gynecology learning and assessment.

For candidates at any OSCE please understand that the OSCE is only less subjective than long cases and other traditional assessment tests. Some subjectivity remains. Although the candidate does not need to wear Dior or Armani, personal hygiene, neatness, appropriate dress and behaviour can only help a candidate's cause to be a future doctor or specialist.

For the undergraduate there is a vital need to become case-hardened with OSCE practice. This book will greatly help. Chapter 1 is most important: many medical students seem unaware how to pace themselves over a 6-minute OSCE station. Time is a fact of life for any modern doctor, whether year 1 or year 25. Please practise your timing and become fluent.

Postgraduates at examinations such as the MRANZCOG or MRCOG must not only be fluent but also clinically mature. History and examination should flow with a rhythm and a cadence rather that like of a concert pianist, over 5 minutes or so. Test yourself, as suggested by Dr Weston and his colleagues, on three or four OSCEs at a time to help become case-hardened and to overcome the 'difficult' station or your odd bad performance. Where you can, try to relate your medical logic and thought processes to the examiner. In postgraduate examinations there may be even more than one OSCE examiner – some colleges have internal checks and audits to root out examiner bias.

An advantage of the OSCE is its easy adaption to many clinical situations – the ward, the operating theatre, the birthing unit or the labour ward. This means examination questions may not be theory from any textbook, but simple things that only a clinical attachment can teach. Writing an operation report or post-operative orders are examples. For many universities this helps focus the medical student on clinical matters in those precious 8 to 10 weeks of their obstetrics and gynecology/women's health course.

My final word of advice is to peak at the right time. All medical students and young doctors are highly intelligent individuals. That is not enough. Athletes for the Olympic Games not only exercise hard, but also eat the world's best food, get proper rest and have focused sports counselling. Medical students and postgraduates should also exercise their bodies as well as their brains, eat well, sleep well and focus to perform at their best. Exhaustion from a part-time job out-of-hours is no preparation for an OSCE.

Professor David Healy
Head, Monash University
Department of Obstetrics and Gynecology

Preface

I hope that medical students and training registrars alike find the practice OSCE exam questions contained in this book valuable in preparing for their respective exams. The questions are designed so that they are undertaken in pairs, with one student acting as the examiner and the other as the exam candidate. There are four sets of eight OSCEs pitched at a medical student level, and a further four sets of eight OSCEs at a MRANZCOG level. My co-authors and I have tried to present questions on a broad range of topics. When attempting to cover the entire specialty it is impossible not to be impressed by the expanse of knowledge contained within obstetrics and gynaecology.

I would like to thank the many teachers who have inspired and taught me much of the art of obstetrics and gynaecology: Professor Ian Pettigrew, Dr John Campbell, Professor David Healy and Dr John Bowditch, to name but a few. To Professor Peter Rogers and Dr Caroline Gargett, a big thank you for teaching me much of the science of obstetrics and gynaecology.

For those of you reading this book and preparing for your exam – good luck!!

Dr Gareth Weston
September 2008

Abbreviations

ACIS	Adenocarcinoma in situ	D&C	Dilatation and currettage
ACL	Anticardiolipin	D&E	Dilatation and evacuation
AFI	Amniotic fluid index	DHEAS	Dehydroepiandrosterone
AFP	Alpha-fetoprotein		sulphate
AIS	Androgen insensitivity	DIC	Disseminated intravascular
	syndrome		coagulation
ANA	Antinuclear antigen	DKA	Diabetic ketoacidosis
APH	Antepartum haemorrhage	DM	Diabetes mellitus
APTT	Activated partial	DNA	Deoxyribose nucleic acid
	thromboplastin time	DVT	Deep venous thrombosis
ARM	Artificial rupture of	ECG	Electrocardiograph
	membranes	EFW	Estimated fetal weight
ASD	Atrial septal defect	Ex	Examination
ASRM	American Society for	FAI	Free androgen index
	Reproductive Medicine	FBE	Full blood examination
Av	Anteverted	FDIU	Fetal death in utero
AXR	Abdominal X-ray	FH(R)	Fetal heart (rate)
BMI	Body mass index	FISH	Fluorescent in situ
BP	Blood pressure		hybridisation
BPM	Beats per minute	FSH	Follicle stimulating
BRCA	Breast cancer gene		hormone
BSL	Blood sugar level	FVL	Factor V Leiden
BSO	Bilateral salpingo-	FWT	Full ward test
	oophorectomy	GBS	Group B streptococcus
CAH	Congenital adrenal	GCT	Glucose challenge test
	hyperplasia	GDM	Gestational diabetes
CEA	Carcinoembryonic antigen	GH	Growth hormone
CF	Cystic fibrosis	GTN	Glyceryl trinitrate
CIN	Cervical intraepithelial	GTT	Glucose tolerance test
	neoplasia	HBV	Hepatitis B virus
CMV	Cytomegalovirus	HCG	Human chorionic
COCP	Combined oral		gonadotrophin
	contraceptive pill	HDL	High density lipoprotein
COGU	Certificate in Obstetrics and	HELLP	Haemolysis, elevated liver
	Gynaecology Ultrasound		enzymes, lowered platelets
CRP	C-reactive protein	HIV	Human immunodeficiency
C/S	Caesarean section		virus
CSE	Combined spinal/epidural	HNPCC	Hereditary non-polyposis
CT	Computerised tomography		colon cancer
CTG	Cardiotocograph	HPV	Human papillomavirus
CVS	Cardiovascular system;	HR	Heart rate
	chorionic villous sampling	HSG	Hysterosalpingogram
CXR	Chest X-ray	HSV	Herpes simplex virus

HT	Hormone therapy	NKA	No known allergies
HVS	High vaginal swab	NVD	Normal vaginal delivery
Hx	History	OA	Occiput anterior
IBT	Immunobead test	OHSS	Ovarian hyperstimulation
ICSI	Intracytoplasmic sperm		syndrome
	injection	OI	Ovulation induction
ICU	Intensive care unit	OT	Operating theatre
IDC	Indwelling catheter	PAI	Plasminogen activation
IDDM	Insulin dependent diabetes		inhibitor
	mellitus	PAP Test	Papanicolaou smear
IGF	Insulin-like growth factor	PAPP	Pregnancy associated
IGT	Impaired glucose tolerance		plasma protein
IM	Intramuscular	PCA	Patient-controlled analgesia
IMB	Intermenstrual bleed	PCB	Postcoital bleed
INR	International normalised	PCOS	Polycystic ovarian
	ratio		syndrome
IUD	Intrauterine device	PCR	Polymerase chain reaction
IUGR	Intrauterine growth	PE	Pulmonary embolus
	retardation	PEEP	Positive end expiratory
IV	Intravenous		pressure
IVDU	IV drug use(r)	PET	Pre-eclamptic toxaemia
IVF	In vitro fertilisation	PHx	Past history
JVP	Jugular venous pressure	PG	Prostaglandin
LAC	Lupus anticoagulant	PGD	Pre-implantation genetic
LBW	Low birth weight		diagnosis
LDH	Lactate dehydrogenase	PID	Pelvic inflammatory disease
LDL	Low density lipoprotein	PO	Per oral
LFT	Liver function test	POC	Products of conception
LH	Luteinising hormone	POD	Pouch of Douglas
LLETZ	Large loop excision of the	POF	Premature ovarian failure
	transformation zone	PPH	Postpartum haemorrhage
LMP	Last menstrual period	PPROM	Preterm premature rupture
LMW	Low molecular weight		of membranes
LUSCS	Lower uterine segment	PR	Pulse rate; per rectum
	caesarean section	PV	Per vagina
LV	Left ventricle	Rh	Rhesus
MCV	Mean cell volume	RIF	Right iliac fossa
MRI	Magnetic resonance	ROM	Rupture of membranes
	imaging	RPR	Rapid plasma reagin
MRKH	Mayer-Rokitansky-	RR	Relative risk; respiratory
	Kuster-Hauser		rate
MSU	Mid-stream urine	RUQ	Right upper quadrant
NHMRC	National Health and	SA	Semen analysis
	Medical Research Council	SCC	Squamous cell carcinoma
NICU	Neonatal intensive care unit	SFH	Symphyseal-fundal height
NIH	National Institutes of	SHBG	Sex-hormone binding
	Health		globulin
NSAIDs	Non-steroidal anti-	SIDS	Sudden infant death
	inflammatory drugs		syndrome

SLE	Systemic lupus erythematosus	TTTS	Twin–twin transfusion syndrome
STD	Sexually transmitted disease	TVT	Tension free vaginal tape
STI	Sexually transmitted infection	U+E+Cr	Urea and electrolytes and creatinine
T	Temperature	U/S	Ultrasound
T21	Trisomy 21	UTI	Urinary tract infection
TENS	Transcutaneous electrical nerve stimulation	VDRL	Venereal disease reference laboratory
TFT	Thyroid function test	VE	Vaginal examination
TOP	Termination of pregnancy	V/Q scan	Ventilation perfusion scan
TORCH	Common transplacental infective organisms	VSD	Ventricular septal defect
		VTE	Venous thromboembolism
TPHA	Treponema pallidum haemagglutination test	WBC	White blood cells
		WCC	White cell count
TSH	Thyroid stimulating hormone	WHI	Women's health initiative
		WHO	World Health Organization

How to approach an OSCE: clinical stations

INTRODUCTION

An 'Objective Structured Clinical Examination' (OSCE) is a short, simulated clinical scenario designed to assess the clinical skills of the examination candidate. This method of examination was first proposed in 1975 by R.M. Harden as one way of providing 'a more objective approach to the assessment of clinical competence'.

In an OSCE examination candidates move through a number of short clinical scenarios which are designed to focus on a range of topics and specific clinical skills. This can be contrasted with the traditional clinical examination – the 'long case' – where the candidate would take a history and examine a patient in private, before presenting examiners with the findings, proposed diagnoses, required investigations and treatment. In his original article, Harden found that the OSCE results had a far better correlation with the written results of the students than the traditional approach as the patient (usually simulated) was the same for all students, while the examiners had a standard marking sheet, making their assessment both clear and reproducible.

Since its introduction the OSCE has become a widely used examination tool for both undergraduate medical student and postgraduate specialist examinations. It is currently a key component of the examination process in Obstetrics and Gynaecology at our institution. While it does not replace the need for written examinations to test purely factual knowledge, it does assess a different range of skills that are of a more practical nature.

Aspects of clinical practice that can be assessed in an OSCE range from taking a patient's general history and asking questions appropriate to the presenting complaint to taking a focused history on a particular problem (such as a menstrual history or a sexual history), explaining investigation results in terms that a patient can understand (e.g. an abnormal fetal ultrasound result or an abnormal Pap smear), performing a specific clinical examination (e.g. a routine newborn examination) or acting out a clinical 'action' such as taking a Pap smear, performing neonatal resuscitation or dealing with a shoulder dystocia in labour.

Medical students

There is often a lot of concern surrounding the OSCEs by medical students as they are less familiar with the format than they are with written examinations, a familiar format first experienced at secondary school. The techniques of history-taking, examination, and counselling and talking to patients are relatively new to them. Nonetheless, these skills are just as important to their future success as doctors as the factual knowledge they gain from reading the textbooks.

MRANZCOG candidates

Candidates for the specialist entry MRANZCOG (Membership of the Royal Australian and New Zealand College of Obstetrics and Gynacology) exam may be more comfortable with history-taking, examining and counselling patients, but less familiar with the OSCE examination process. While the exams aim to mimic clinical practice, there is a certain 'knack' to passing them which requires an understanding of their format and how they are assessed.

The importance of practice

The old saying that 'repetition is the mother of learning' is no less true of OSCEs than it is of any other examination type. There is no doubt that the more practice cases and scenarios candidates experience, the more likely they are to pass the exam. This textbook has been written with the aim of providing a significant number of practice cases, together with a detailed marking scheme, so that exam candidates working in pairs will be able to assess each other objectively and improve their performance by reviewing ideal answers. Not all examination candidates manage to obtain enough practice before the OSCE exam, and the preparation of cases by 'practice' examiners is time-consuming, meaning that busy doctors are often unable to provide adequate time to go through practice cases. We hope that this book will allow candidates for an OSCE in Obstetrics and Gynaecology, either at undergraduate or postgraduate level, to gain sufficient practice before the exam to maximise their chances of a pass.

BASIC OSCE STRUCTURE

Medical students

The basic structure of OSCEs for medical students may vary from institution to institution, and you should check with your faculty to see what your institution expects. At our university OSCEs are usually made up of 1 minute reading time, followed by 6 minutes with the examiner, often with an actor playing the role of the patient. After the first 5 minutes (i.e. after 6 minutes of the 7-minute station), the examiner is required to give an indication to the candidate that only 1 minute remains before the end of the OSCE station. At the end of the 7 minutes a bell is sounded and the examination candidate must move on to the next station.

MRANZCOG candidates

The MRANZCOG OSCEs have a uniform format for all candidates. At present the OSCEs are 20 minutes in total, with 5 minutes reading time at the start of the station, followed by 15 minutes with the examiner. Obviously these OSCEs are more complex than the cases for the medical students, and the candidates often have three to five scenarios to go through, which test a wide range of both obstetric and gynaecological knowledge before they can proceed to the next station. Generally at the first station the candidate takes a detailed history from the simulated patient (either an actor or the examiner playing the role of the patient and answering questions).

Marking

The OSCE examiner usually has a marking sheet with a set of marks assigned to key clinical points – either specific questions relating to history, examinations performed, differential diagnoses, or information on prognosis or implications for the patient's health imparted to the patient. This rather rigid marking scheme means that marks can be gained only for the specific points indicated. However, it does ensure a uniform marking scheme for all examination candidates, allowing for the marks of two candidates to be directly compared.

One problem that arises with this marking scheme is that some candidates demonstrate more orderly and logical thought processes in the way that they direct history-taking, examination and investigation of the patient than others. Therefore, some OSCEs will have a proportion of marks assigned to 'clinical competency' (e.g. 5 out of 20 marks), so that well-organised candidates have the opportunity to distinguish themselves.

Reading time

Reading time is an integral part of the OSCE, and it is very important to use this time wisely. It is even more important in the MRANZCOG OSCE, as there are 5 minutes assigned, rather than the 1 minute allocated for the medical student OSCE. The amount to be 'read' may only amount to one or two sentences, but there is important information in those few short lines. The introductory information may be presented, for example, as a letter from a referring general practitioner, or as a short clinical description.

Extracting maximum information from the introduction

EXAMPLE: Mrs Bloggs is a 41- year-old G3 P2 at 8/40 gestation presenting for her first antenatal visit.

This introduction has already given us a number of pieces of important information. First, the patient's age – she is 41 years old and of advanced maternal age. She will need to be counselled about the increased risk of miscarriage (due to aneuploidy), gestational diabetes in pregnancy (she will need a glucose tolerance test rather than just a glucose challenge test at 28/40), pre-eclampsia and Down syndrome (one in 100 risk – need to discuss screening/amniocentesis/chorionic villous sampling).

Second, she has had two previous deliveries of greater than 20 weeks gestation. We will need to ask about the mode of delivery, the gestation at delivery and any previous pregnancy, delivery (e.g. shoulder dystocia), or post-delivery problems (e.g. post-partum haemorrhage, breastfeeding problems, Group-B streptococcal infections in the neonates). All of these pieces of information may impact on our management of the pregnancy.

Third, the patient is at 8 weeks gestation, so issues to be encountered are likely to occur, at least initially, in the first trimester. We will need to ask about early pregnancy problems (e.g. bleeding, pain, hyperemesis gravidarum, urinary problems). Finally, we are told that the patient is presenting for her first antenatal visit, so we will need to order and explain all of the routine antenatal screening (FBE, blood group and antibodies, rubella IgG levels, hepatitis B serology, RPR or other test for syphilis, offer HIV testing, midstream urine for culture, and possibly a first trimester ultrasound for dating the pregnancy).

Most of the introductory scenarios will similarly have information to be gleaned to a greater or lesser degree (see the boxed text below for common clinical points from the introductory statement). Use the reading time to jot down as much of the information or relevant history and examination details as you can, so that you remember it. It is easy to forget a seemingly minor detail that becomes very important to the scenario later on.

Common points of information in the introductory statement

- Age of patient:

Young patients (<21)
- Social/financial difficulties
- Recreational drugs
- Increased risk of STDs (esp chlamydia), consider screening if appropriate
- Contraception, Pap smears

Older women (>38)
- Increased risk of Down syndrome in pregnancies
- Reduced fertility with increasing age, increased miscarriage risk
- Increased risk of gestational diabetes and pre-eclampsia (in pregnancies)

Post-menopausal
- Increased risk of osteoporosis, menopausal symptoms, cancers, prolapse, urinary incontinence and sexual problems (vaginal atrophy, reduced libido); ask regarding mammograms

BMI (>30)
- Counsel regarding diet/exercise
- General health issues (heart disease, arthritis, sleep apnoea, blood cholesterol, etc)
- Specific gynae and obstetric issues (increased risk of gestational diabetes, miscarriage, PCOS, operative risks, etc)

BMI (<18)
- Hypothalamic/pituitary anovulation if eating disorder
- Ask regarding diet (adequate?) and exercise (excessive?)

Presenting clinical problem
- Need to focus on this and address first in history

Gestation
- Consider questions/conditions relevant to gestation

Parity
- Consider effects of parity on current gynae/obstetric problem

Aboriginal
- Social/financial difficulties; domestic violence?
- Alcohol and drug-related issues
- Cultural sensitivity/Aboriginal liaison officer to be involved

Intravenous drug-user
- HepB, HepC, HIV screen; liver function if HBV or HCV +ve
- Effects of drugs on pregnancies (e.g. IUGR, neonatal dependence, risk of abruption or FDIU)
- Social/financial issues

Sex worker
- Social/financial issues
- Recreational drugs
- Sexually transmitted diseases/PID

Be organised

Adopting an organised approach to extracting clinical information from the 'patient', and addressing the clinical problems presented are crucial to your success in the OSCE. In the MRANZCOG (and in most medical student) exams, candidates are allowed to write notes on a blank sheet of paper, both during the reading time and during the examination time with the examiner. The candidates at our institution have an extremely high success rate, in part due to adopting a systematic approach to note-making. While there are any number of ways of organising your notes, below is one effective suggestion.

Divide the paper into three columns (see Figure 1.1). In the first column list in logical order aspects of the history you wish to ask the 'patient'. In the second column list aspects of the examination you wish to perform. In the third column list investigations and management, which will usually be dictated by information in the history or examination. For example, if the patient is a smoker you would list this in the history column and then draw a line across to management and ask for a CXR/lung function test (if working up for a gynaecological operation), counsel about the dangers of smoking to the woman's health (including fertility), as well as that of her unborn baby (if pregnant or trying to get pregnant), or of her child (e.g. risk of SIDS if she has an infant at home).

At the bottom of the page an 'Issues list' can be drawn up, so that issues identified during the reading time or the history-taking are not forgotten later on when counselling the patient. Remember, the examiner has a tick list of clinical information to be gleaned from the patient when assigning your marks, and you want to get as many of these as possible. Good techniques at this stage will maximise your OSCE marks, helping you through the stage when you will probably be feeling at your most nervous and flustered.

An ordered approach to history-taking and examination points

An organised candidate for the OSCE exam will use an ordered approach when taking a gynaecological and obstetric history, as well as when asking for points on examination. You will not usually be expected to actually perform an examination (it would be impossible for a simulated patient to endure 20 to 30 pelvic examinations), but you will be expected to know precisely what examinations you would like to perform.

The candidate then asks for the results of their examination. If you fail to ask for particular examinations to be performed the examiner will not reveal the examination findings, which may be crucial to the management of the patient. Thus, it is important to make sure that you approach the

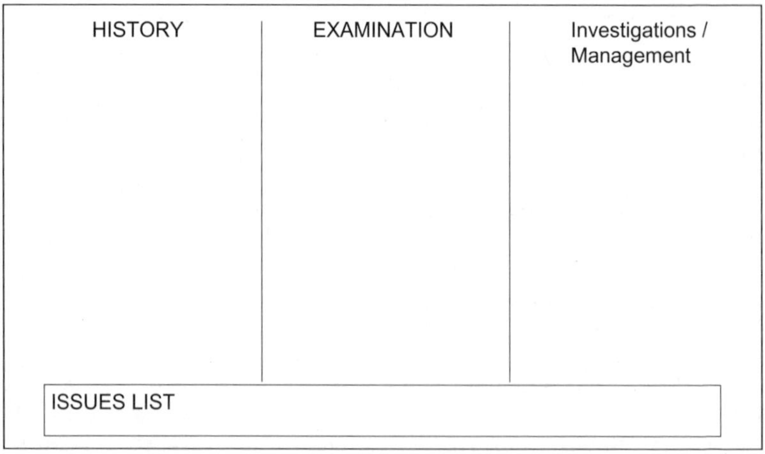

HISTORY	EXAMINATION	Investigations / Management

ISSUES LIST

Figure 1.1   An effective method for note-taking

history and examination in a thorough manner. Practice OSCEs help to get candidates into a routine where they are more likely to remember the key points of history and examination they should be asking for during the actual OSCE examination, when stress levels are at their highest.

Two important points to note about taking the initial history examination are: first, be thorough but efficient; and second, adjust the type and order of questions to address the particular presenting problem.

Be thorough but efficient
Medical students
In a medical student exam, time management is critical. There will often be several marks assigned to extra questions at the end of the OSCE case. Often candidates spend far too long on the initial history and examination phase. While they may get the majority of the marks for the first station of the OSCE, they will get an overall low mark because they have not been able to attempt the marks assigned to the later questions.

MRANZCOG candidates
There are likely to be up to five to six scenarios to pass through in a single MRANZCOG OSCE station. Therefore, it is important to leave enough time to actually get through all of the scenarios.

Possible approaches – all candidates
Split questions on history or examination into groups (no more than three at a time), and ask for two to three aspects of history or examination at once to save time. Be careful not to lump too many questions together, especially if they are potentially complex, to avoid confusing the examiner/simulated patient. Speak quickly, but not so fast as to render your questions unintelligible to the examiner. If they cannot understand what you have said they might miss it altogether and you will not get marks for the knowledge you have displayed. This last point is especially important for exam candidates from non-English-speaking backgrounds – speak clearly and practise with native English speakers if possible to ensure you can be understood on exam day. Don't ask too many extraneous questions, such as aspects of history already given in the introduction, and keep questions designed to look for specific rare diagnoses to a minimum. While demonstrating your knowledge of relevant differential diagnoses, an exhaustive number of questions on rare conditions will eat into your examination time and are less likely to have marks assigned to them.

Addressing the presenting problem
It displays poor clinical acumen if the candidate blindly recites a long list of questions on history and examination without making any reference to the particular problem. The examiner is looking for a future clinician, not a robot. If the scenario is a gynaecological one, start with the gynae history first, and then ask for the past obstetric history, and vice versa. Take

a more detailed history regarding the presenting complaint, but less detail with regard to aspects of gynae/obstetric history that is not relevant to the particular scenario presented.

Think carefully when asking for aspects of examination. If the patient is a 17-year-old girl who has not had sexual intercourse, do not blunder into asking for a vaginal examination. If the patient is a 50-year-old woman who has a past history of a hysterectomy, do not ask for a Pap smear! The effective candidate not only has a rough outline or approach to their history and examination, but can think on their feet so that the condition of the actual patient represented in the scenario is considered at all times. After all, this is exactly what happens in real-life clinical practice.

Suggested templates for gynae and obstetric initial encounters are presented over the next three pages.

History/examination of the gynae patient

(Questions that should be grouped together are listed on the same line.)

History

- Patient name and age
- Presenting complaint: what is the primary reason the patient presents today?
- Menstrual history:
  - Age at menarche/menopause
  - How many days since last menstrual period?
  - Are cycles regular? How many days does she bleed? Average length of cycles
- Are periods heavy? (if so, how long has it been present? Clots/flooding? How many pads used per day? Has she had any previous treatments? If so, how effective were they? Side effects?)
- Are periods painful? (if so, when during cycle? How does it affect daily functioning – e.g. number of days off work? Any treatments? Effective? Side effects?)
- Any intermenstrual bleeding? Post-coital bleeding? Post-menopausal bleeding?
- Sexually active at present? Any problems with intercourse? Dyspareunia? (If so, timecourse, and whether superficial or deep, or related to cycles)
- Contraception – types tried, failures/unwanted pregnancies, side effects
- Vaginal discharge (If present: colour, odour, itch, irritation?); past history; sexually transmitted diseases? (If so, treated? Contact tracing? Checked for other STDs?)
- Last Pap smear? Does she have regular Pap smears? (What frequency?) Normal? Ever abnormal? (If so, what treatment?)
- Last mammogram/breast ultrasound?
- Menopausal symptoms (if age-appropriate, or amenorrhoea)

- Urinary incontinence/symptoms; prolapse/lump in vagina; bowel symptoms
- Pelvic pain (not associated with menses or intercourse)
- Past gynaecological history: past diagnoses (and basis for diagnosis), past operations
- Past obstetric history (see obstetric history-taking for details)
- Past medical history; past psychiatric history
- Past surgical history
- Family history (of cancers, or medical and genetic conditions)
- Social history: home, relationships, work, financial/social stresses
- Smoking history; alcohol intake; other recreational drugs
- Medications; allergies

Examination
- General appearance (colour, secondary sexual characteristics)
- Vitals (temperature, blood pressure, pulse rate, respiratory rate); body mass index; full ward test (urine pregnancy test if appropriate)
  - *(remember: inspection, palpation, percussion, auscultation)*
- Thyroid, cardio-respiratory and breast examination
- Abdominal examination
- Inspection of external genitalia (lumps, skin conditions, ulcers, discolouration, atrophy), including urethral meatus
- Bimanual examination: Uterine size and shape; anteverted/retroverted; tenderness; mobility; adnexal masses
- Joint vaginal and rectal examination (if appropriate – for Pouch of Douglas nodules/tenderness)

Speculum examination
- Bi-valve to inspect vaginal walls and cervix (take Pap smears and high vaginal/cervical swabs if appropriate)
- Sims speculum to examine for prolapse (systematically examine anterior and posterior vaginal wall then vault) and urinary incontinence (loss of urine with cough).

History/examination of the obstetric patient: Antenatal history

- Patient name and age

Current pregnancy
- Spontaneous or assisted conception (IVF/ovulation induction; reason for infertility)
- Planned pregnancy? Wanted pregnancy?
- Gestation: last menstrual period (gestation by dates); if by ultrasound, when performed and findings (nuchal translucency, singleton/twins, placenta, other findings, e.g. fibroid, ovarian cyst)

- On folate or multivitamins prior to conception? Rubella/parvovirus/varicella checked prior to conception?
- Current pregnancy symptoms (ask appropriate to gestation: first trimester – hyperemesis, breast tenderness, urinary Sx; third trimester – backache, gastro-oesophageal reflux)
- Any screening Ix performed to date? What results?

Past obstetric history
- Pregnancies in order with their outcomes
- Early pregnancy losses: miscarriages (gestation, treatment, complications); terminations (gestation, mode of TOP, complications); ectopics (type, gestation, treatment)
- Pregnancies > 20/40 (gestation at delivery; medical complications of previous pregnancies; mode of delivery; delivery complications – post-partum haemorrhage, shoulder dystocia; puerperal complications – infections, breast-feeding issues, postnatal depression)
- Gynaecological and general history as above, but with less comprehensive questioning of gynaecological history

Examination
- General history is as above for gynaecological history, until the candidate reaches the abdominal examination
- N.B. Check urine for protein and glucose on dipstick
- Abdominal and vaginal examination depending on gestation

First trimester
- Abdominal/vaginal Ex: Is uterus palpable abdominally? If not, what size uterus on vaginal examination? Speculum for Pap smear if due

Second trimester/third trimester
- Abdominal Ex: symphyseal-fundal height (SFH); lie and presentation of fetus; single or multiple pregnancy; doppler of fetal heart (present? rate?); miscellaneous findings (fibroid, uterine tenderness)
- Vaginal Ex (only if appropriate)
  - Cervical length, dilatation, consistency, position, station of presenting part

---

History/examination of the obstetric patient: Intrapartum history

- Patient name and age
- Parity
- Single or multiple pregnancy
- Mode of previous deliveries; prior delivery complications
- Brief medical/surgical history
- Medications (including syntocinon), allergies

- Presenting complaint (often called by midwife/junior doctor)
- Progress of labour (contractions, vaginal assessments)
- Status of membranes, colour of liquor
- Use of analgesia (pethidine? How long ago? epidural?)
- Assessment of fetal wellbeing (fetal heart rate, CTG)

Examination
- General: BP, full ward test of urine, pulse rate, temperature
- Abdominal Ex: Lie, presentation, SFH, fetal heart, contractions
- Vaginal Ex: Presentation, station, position, moulding, caput; cervix–dilatation, length, position; assessment of pelvis

   N.B. *This is likely to be a more fast-paced encounter focusing on management of emergencies and the history needs to be abbreviated to focus on the crucial issues that pose a risk to the mother and fetus(es). For example, make sure that this is not a trial of scar, a placenta praevia, multiple pregnancy or a breech presentation. Check for gestational diabetes, hypertension, anaemia or concerns regarding IUGR. Exclude significant maternal illnesses such as type 1 diabetes, asthma, epilepsy, stroke or cardiac disease.*

WRAPPING IT UP

After taking a detailed but appropriate history and examination, there will usually be a number of investigations and/or aspects of management or treatment to be initiated. The better candidates will end the first scenario with a list of problems or issues. Rather than just listing a lot of investigations and treatments, they will be linked to the issues identified. Never simply state that you wish an investigation to be performed, but state *why* the investigation is needed (i.e. what you are looking for). This lets the examiner know that you are thinking about the clinical case, and that you understand why you need to perform the investigations.

If you are recommending invasive investigations and/or treatments, you should be prepared to immediately mention possible risks of surgery or side effects of medications. There are significant time pressures in an OSCE, so you should interact with the examiner or simulated patient by asking them if they would like you to go into more detail. A statement such as: "There are potential complications of this surgery. Would you like me to discuss these in detail with you?", is a good start. If it is not important to the particular scenario or there are no marks attached to it in the marking scheme the examiner may indicate that it is unnecessary to avoiding time-wasting.

Medical students

For medical student OSCEs there is generally only one scenario, unless your institution has longer OSCE times – 6 minutes is simply not long enough to allow for multiple complex encounters, but it is enough to allow for a series of further related questions.

To wrap up the scenario for a medical student we would suggest aiming to spend 2 minutes on history-taking and 1 minute on the examination.

MRANZCOG candidates

As the first scenario is the first of several for a MRANZCOG OSCE, wrapping it up in a timely fashion is critical to having enough time to secure the marks assigned to the later scenarios. We would suggest trying to aim for 3 minutes for the history-taking, with a further 2 minutes for the examination in a MRANZCOG OSCE. Obviously there will be some stations where this will not be possible, so this is only a rough guide.

MOVING ON: FURTHER ENCOUNTERS OF THE OSCE KIND
MRANZCOG candidates

In the MRANZCOG OSCEs there will usually be further clinical encounters. For example, you may have further encounters with an obstetric patient at different stages of gestation. A gynae patient may become pregnant for a later encounter. You may encounter the patient before, during and after surgery, with a different set of clinical problems to be identified and managed at each scenario.

It is important *not* to assume that the clinical issues in the first encounter are to be the only ones for the entire OSCE. The issues can suddenly change from one encounter to the next. Always start each new encounter within a single OSCE station with an open mind and ask for a brief, fresh history and examination. If you forget to check on changes to history and examination in the same patient at different encounters you may miss important changes to the patient's condition. Also be careful not to forget aspects of history or examination from the first encounter which may not become important until the third or fourth encounter. For example, there may have been a family history of breast cancer discovered in the first encounter which only becomes important when discussing the possible use of hormone therapy in the final encounter. Alternatively, a patient's past history of a midline laparotomy from a burst appendix may only become important when considering performing a laparoscopy in the final encounter, necessitating a Hassan entry rather than a Veress needle, or a Palmers point entry rather than umbilical. Being able to refer to an issues list jotted down from the reading time and first encounter will minimise your chance of forgetting these key aspects of history and examination points in the later encounters.

Remember that it is not necessary to be brilliant in each encounter during an OSCE station in order to pass the station. It is possible that you may mess up one encounter. Try not to let that affect your subsequent encounters. Keep moving through the encounters trying to extract as many marks as possible from each. Almost all of the candidates for the OSCE exam will do badly in some of their encounters – you will not be the only one. It is also possible that you may run out of time before completing all of the encounters or questions for the station. Again, this does not mean you have failed the station overall. Put it behind you and move on to the next station with a clear and calm head.

There are a number of particular types of questions in further encounters of the OSCEs that you can have prepared answers for. Many past MRANZCOG OSCEs have had questions asking candidates to describe how to perform a particular procedure (e.g. a forceps delivery, a gynaecological operation, and so on). Memorise a logical description of all common gynaecology and obstetric procedures, including positioning of the patient, prepping and draping, type of incision, short description of the surgical steps of the procedure, risks and steps to minimise the risks. Do not be exhaustive in your description, but emphasise key points. There are only likely to be a small number of marks assigned to the encounter. Examples of other questions you can have a prepared answer for include: describe types of electrosurgical injuries; describe how to locate and ligate the internal iliac arteries; describe how to perform an external cephalic version, or contraindications for vaginal birth after caesarean section.

It is important to practise discussing consent for medical treatments, procedures and/or surgery – particularly risks and possible complications. For example, if a candidate prescribes clomiphene citrate for anovulatory infertility but does not mention side effects or the risk of multiple pregnancy (and why multiple pregnancy is an undesirable outcome!), they have not fully informed the patient and may miss marks assigned to these points in the encounter.

GENERAL PREPARATION TIPS FOR AN OSCE

All candidates

This text aims to provide OSCE examination candidates with a number of practice scenarios. Practise as many as you can prior to the examination. Try to cover all aspects of the gynaecology/obstetrics syllabus. Also try to cover a large number of possible different formats, such as phone-call advice, emergency management, regular clinical encounters in outpatient settings, post-natal and post-operative complications, grief counselling, and dealing with angry or emotional patients. This will minimise your chance of being 'thrown' by an encounter format on the day of the examination. If there are published past examination questions for your OSCE, then practise those as well. Contact your mentors for face-to-face practice cases. It is a good idea to perform three or four practice OSCEs per week leading up to your examination. If you can form a study group with fellow candidates this will improve your practice as you will be able to observe other people practising OSCEs and thereby get tips of both what to do and what not to do.

Examiners are trained not to give any clues to the candidate as to how they are going in the exam. Do not expect encouragement from the examiner and do not feel you are doing badly if they do not show any sign that you are doing well. If the examiner signals that you should move on to other issues in your wrapping up of the first encounter, don't keep reciting your knowledge. It is likely that they are trying to time-manage the OSCE to give you enough time for the further stations. Some candidates get frustrated that they have been unable to demonstrate all of their knowledge, but it is no use demonstrating knowledge for which there are no marks assigned in the station – better to move on to further encounters in the station with marks assigned to them.

In some OSCE stations you will finish with time to spare. This does not necessarily mean that you have missed information – some of the OSCEs may be shorter than others. It can be unnerving to have to sit there in silence for a minute in an OSCE. Try to think if there are any issues you have missed during the station, and discuss them. There may still be marks to be had. During a MRANZCOG OSCE, however, you may only gain marks by discussing matters relevant to the last encounter of the OSCE. The rules regarding medical student OSCEs will vary from institution to institution.

You must remember to list even the most simple or obvious things that may appear to be second nature to you; for example, stating the regular antenatal visits to an obstetric patient and the health checks performed at each antenatal visit. It is easy to forget to state the obvious (e.g. 'monochorionic diamniotic twin pregnancy is a high-risk pregnancy').

It is also easy to forget to state exactly what you want done for a patient admitted to the ward. Many candidates fall into the trap of assuming that management decisions will be made by others, as is common in a team approach to public patients. This is not the case in the OSCE. You cannot assume that the patient's blood pressure and temperature will be checked or that the drain-tube output will be measured, unless you specifically ask for it. You should also set limits at which you wish to be contacted (such as an upper limit of blood pressure in a pre-eclamptic patient, an upper limit of blood sugar level in a diabetic patient or a lower limit of oxygen saturation in a patient with ovarian hyperstimulation syndrome, in case pleural effusions develop). You must treat your description of management for a patient as though you are instructing staff who have never seen the particular condition before. After all, in the examination it is important to demonstrate that *you* know how to instruct regarding regular observations for your patients.

When considering management approaches for a patient in a clinical scenario, always think in a conservative fashion. Choose the safest, most careful course of action. If in doubt, admit the patient for observation and investigation. It is better to be safe and cautious than take risks with the patient's care.

Try to be engaging with the simulated patient, and appropriate (i.e. serious when discussing complications or grief-counselling, bright and cheerful when taking a history). Do not crack jokes with the patient or examiner – this will not make you look like a competent clinician and may offend the patient. Ask for permission before performing invasive examinations, such as vaginal or rectal examinations. You would not perform these without permission in real life, and should mimic this in your OSCE.

Finally, we wish you good luck, and hope that the practice exam questions contained in this text help you to successfully prepare for your OSCE examination.

2

How to approach an OSCE: counselling stations

INTRODUCTION

Some OSCEs are designed to concentrate more on candidates' counselling skills than on their display of medical and technical knowledge. In our interactions with patients in real life, counselling skills are often just as important – and sometimes more important – than our ability to recite medical facts and figures as we tell them what treatment they might need.

The counselling stations allow the examiner to get a sense of how you speak and communicate with patients. Some examples of situations when counselling skills are tested include: the delivery of bad news; dealing with an angry or upset patient; and explaining a complex clinical problem, and/or treatment, to a patient in terms they can understand.

DELIVERY OF BAD NEWS

'Bad news' can be defined as any information which radically and negatively alters the patient's perception about their own future. While it is most commonly associated with the diagnosis of a terminal illness, such as ovarian cancer, in the context of obstetrics and gynaecology it may be the loss of a baby (e.g. fetal death in utero diagnosed on a scan), or the loss of reproductive potential (e.g. a hysterectomy performed to control bleeding in a young woman, or the discovery that a young woman has Turner's syndrome and has gone through premature menopause, so will be unable to have children naturally). The patient experiences a perceived loss (i.e. of life-span, of a baby, or of reproductive potential), and will go through a variable grief reaction.

Kubler-Ross identified the five stages of the grief reaction to death and dying (denial, anger, bargaining, depression, acceptance), which can easily be applied to any grief reaction by a patient. While the short duration of an OSCE does not fully reflect the reality of dealing with bad news (it will usually take much longer, and multiple consultations with the patient), it is worth remembering some basic counselling skills which may help in an OSCE where the delivery of bad news is assessed.

When the candidate knows that bad news must be delivered it is important to try to prepare the patient before delivering it. Identify yourself to the patient, and to any other family members present. Offer to have family members present, if appropriate (e.g. a husband or partner if a fetal death in utero has occurred; a mother or father if a young girl has been diagnosed with a serious congenital reproductive problem).

The patient should be warned that bad news is about to be delivered, so that they can prepare themselves; for example, "I am sorry to say that I have some bad news from the results of your tests", or "I am afraid that the results of the ultrasound scan are not good". It is important that you are empathic in the manner in which you deliver the bad news, and that you indicate from your manner that you care about the patient's reaction to the news and take the situation very seriously.

The bad news must be delivered clearly and slowly, avoiding the use of technical medical terms. You will need to pause at times to ask the patient if they have understood what you have just explained, and be prepared to ask them if they have any questions about the information you have imparted. Offer to provide written material, if necessary. Also consider the emotional impact of bad news and offer professional counselling, further visits to re-explain things, and patient support groups and resources if appropriate and available. Colleagues should never be criticised when delivering bad news, even when it is perceived that the negative outcome is related to their action or inaction, as this will not help the patient in their immediate situation.

Once the bad news has been imparted in a clear and sensitive manner, it is important to explain what medical intervention is needed to deal with the problem (e.g. possible induction of labour for a fetal death in utero; an operation for ovarian cancer). Before moving on to explaining treatment and prognosis, ask the patient if they are ready for you to continue. Again, explain your possible management strategies in a clear and sensitive manner, and give realistic information about their prognosis.

Finally, it is not uncommon for patients to be dealing with feelings of guilt surrounding negative clinical outcomes, particularly where miscarriage or death of a fetus is concerned. It is important to acknowledge this, and, where possible, to anticipate these feelings by addressing them directly. For example, when counselling a woman with a miscarriage, as part of a routine explanation make a point of informing the patient that the miscarriage has not been caused by her working during early pregnancy or by sexual activity. The patient often harbours feelings of guilt that these actions may have played a role in causing the miscarriage.

DEALING WITH AN ANGRY OR UPSET PATIENT

During your OSCE there will often be times when the patient may be distressed or angry about the clinical situation they find themselves in. One common scenario will be a patient with a post-operative complication. There are many such examples in the OSCEs in this text.

In real-life practice, patients should be clearly informed before a procedure of any possible complications, and the chances that they may occur. Without this, informed consent has not been obtained. If a patient is warned about possible complications beforehand they are far less likely to be angry with you about them afterwards, and are far less likely to initiate litigation proceedings. Similarly, in your OSCE, when discussing possible treatments it should be routine to offer to discuss potential complications if they proceed with treatment.

If a negative outcome occurs during treatment of a patient in an OSCE you must not be evasive about the problem. Explain clearly what has happened and how it has happened. It is important to express regret that the complication has occurred and good practice to say 'sorry' to the patient.

It is vital to have a clear plan of how to deal with the problem after you have identified it and explained it to the patient. The patient might display considerable anger. Do not talk over them; allow them to express their anger, acknowledge their feelings. For example, you could say: "I can see that you are angry about the situation, and that is perfectly understandable."

Once the situation has been explained, and the patient's feelings acknowledged, the candidate should outline a clear plan of action. The patient will regain confidence in a clinician who can demonstrate that they not only know what has gone wrong but what can be done about it. This ends the consultation on a positive note, for example: "It is regrettable that this has happened, but now we know what is wrong with you, and this is what we can do to fix it", or "It is unfortunate that this has happened this time, but now this is what we can do to prevent this happening again".

EXPLAINING COMPLEX CLINICAL PROBLEMS AND TREATMENTS

Some OSCEs will involve the diagnosis of a condition with wide-ranging and complex clinical consequences for the patient. For example, polycystic ovarian syndrome has a range of implications for the patient: reproductive potential (anovulation), hyperandrogenism (acne and hisutism), and long-term clinical consequences (obesity, hypercholesterolaemia, diabetes, endometrial cancer risk). It is easy to lose the patient in the details unless the issues are dealt with in an orderly fashion.

Divide the issues up and deal with them one at a time. You may choose to deal with the most serious issues first or with the issue that has caused their presentation to you. With each clinical problem, outline in lay terms what the clinical problems are, how they can be monitored or investigated, and any available treatments for them. Many conditions have both short-term and long-term associated problems. The patient will usually want to know about the short-term implications of their condition first, followed by the long-term problems.

Some scenarios will present a clinical problem and expect you to counsel the patient about treatment options. Again, it is important to strike a balance between imparting information (you want to demonstrate to the examiner that you have the medical knowledge), and making it understandable to the patient.

When describing an array of medical treatments it is important to have an organised framework. Not only does this make it clearer to the patient, but it makes it less likely that you will forget any available interventions. Below is a list of types of treatment, starting from less invasive to more invasive:

- General measures
- Exercises/physiotherapy
- Medical treatments
  - Tablets
  - Injections
  - Medicated devices
- Surgical treatments
  - Minor surgery
  - Major surgery

Not all categories will be appropriate for all situations, but if you run through these headings mentally during the delivery of your answer you will be unlikely to forget any treatment options. For example, when counselling a patient regarding treatment options for menorrhagia:

- General measures: iron tablets/vitamin C tablets
- Exercises/physiotherapy: not appropriate
- Medical treatments
  - Tablets: tranexamic acid; oral contraceptive pill; NSAIDs; progestagen
  - Injections: Depo Provera
  - Medicated devices: Mirena IUD
- Surgical treatments
  - Minor surgery: endometrial ablation/resection
  - Major surgery: hysterectomy

Remember not only to describe the treatments simply and clearly, but any side effects and complications that could arise from various medications or surgery. Also, explain why some treatments may not be appropriate for the particular patient presented in the OSCE (e.g. surgical options for menorrhagia inappropriate for a 16-year-old girl; the oral contraceptive pill not appropriate for a woman with a past history of several episodes of deep venous thrombosis).

CONCLUSION

In an OSCE where counselling is a major feature it is likely that there will be fewer scenarios, as counselling requires more time than simply outlining medical management. Even in an OSCE where counselling is not a major feature, the good candidate will display some of the above principles in their interaction with the role-playing patient.

There are as many types of possible OSCE counselling scenarios as there are possible clinical interactions with patients in real-life practice. The best preparation for counselling in an OSCE is undoubtedly honing clinical counselling skills in clinics and hospital wards while dealing with real patients.

3

Practice OSCE questions for medical student exams

STUDENT OSCE A

A1 **Q1**

Mrs Brown is a 24-year-old nullipara with a 20-year history of type 1 diabetes (insulin-dependent diabetes mellitus). She wishes to have a baby. Please take a history and counsel.

Q2

Please counsel Mrs Brown with respect to pregnancy planning and care based on the history you have obtained.

A2 **Q1**

You are a rural GP obstetrician called by the midwives. "Mrs Wyatt delivered her baby 15 minutes ago, and is now bleeding very heavily. Could you please come to the labour ward as soon as possible."

Describe your assessment and management of the patient.

Q2

What are the risk factors for a post-partum haemorrhage? (In general – not specific to this patient.)

Q3

Would this episode change your management of Mrs Wyatt's labour for her next baby? If so, how?

A3 **Q1**

You are attached to the Gynaecology Oncology Unit and have just assisted at a laparotomy on a 54-year-old woman with advanced ovarian cancer. She has had a total abdominal hysterectomy, bilateral salpingo-oophorectomy and omentectomy. Blood loss was estimated at 300 mL and 5 L of ascitic fluid was drained at the time of the surgery. Fluid replacement was 2.5 L crystalloid and urine output was 250 mL.

Please describe your post-operative orders for the first 24 hours. The patient is stable; there are no drains in situ. The patient has an indwelling urinary catheter and has patient-controlled analgesia (PCA) with morphine.

Q2

It is day 3 post-op. The patient has been stable and was commenced on clear fluids yesterday. You are asked to see her as she has vomited a large volume of bile-stained fluid and is complaining of abdominal pain.

Please assess the patient.

Q3

What investigations would you like to order?

Q4

The results of the investigations are as follows:
- CXR: mild atelectasis only
- AXR: air-fluid levels and distended loops of small bowel
- FBE: Hb 10.6 g/dl, WCC 18.0
- Urea/electrolytes: potassium 3.0, otherwise normal

What is your diagnosis and management?

A4 Mr and Mrs F are unable to become pregnant after trying for 3 years. Please advise.

Q1

Please take a history about the presenting problem.

Q2

Please ask for relevant examination findings.

Q3

What are the key investigations to be performed?

A5 Q1

You are seeing Ms Veronica Hilton, a 23-year-old woman who wishes to try to have a baby in the next few months. She smokes 20 cigarettes a day and drinks 2–3 glasses of wine a night.

You are speaking to the patient. Please counsel her about the risks of smoking and alcohol, with particular reference to obstetric and gynaecological problems.

Q2

Ms Hilton is now 12 weeks pregnant, and has stopped drinking alcohol. However, she still smokes 10 cigarettes a day.

"Can I use nicotine patches to help me stop smoking, doctor?"

Q3

Ms Hilton has a friend who doesn't smoke or drink, but uses cocaine at parties and is 20 weeks pregnant.

"Can cocaine harm her pregnancy, doctor?"

A6 **Q1**

You are seeing Mrs Prouse, a 70-year-old woman with three episodes of vaginal bleeding over the last 6 weeks.

Please take a history from Mrs Prouse.

Q2

What examination findings would you like to know?

Q3

What are the most appropriate investigations?

Q4

What features are you looking for in the ultrasound scan?

Q5

The curettings show a grade 1 endometrioid adenocarcinoma. What is the most appropriate treatment for Mrs Prouse's cancer?

A7 **Q1**

Miss Bertram is a 23-year-old woman who has come to see you following her routine Pap smear. The Pap smear has shown low-grade cervical dysplasia – CIN1/HPV.

Please explain this to her, as well as your management plan.

Q2

Is there a role for the HPV vaccine in this woman?

Q3

Describe the HPV vaccines currently available.

Q4

Miss Bertram returns in 12 months for her repeat Pap smear, which still shows CIN1/HPV. What is the next course of action?

Q5

What does a colposcopy involve?

Q6

Miss Bertram has a biopsy that shows CIN3/HPV. The transformation zone is in full view, and the changes do not extend up the endocervical canal. What are the treatment options?

A8 **Q1**

Ms H, a 24-year-old woman, presents to you complaining of pelvic pain. Please manage her problem.

Q2

Ms H's abdominal and pelvic examination found a normal sized uterus which was fixed in a retroverted position. There was the impression of a mass on the right side of the pelvis.

Ms H has a laparoscopy at which endometriosis is seen and the areas of endometriosis are removed. Please explain endometriosis to Ms H and the management of her condition.

STUDENT OSCE B

B1 **Q1**

Ms V is presenting for the 'morning-after pill'. She had unprotected sex last night with a long-standing male partner.

Please take a history from Ms V.

Q2

Please inform Ms V on the different types of emergency contraception currently available in Australia, their effectiveness and side effects.

Q3

What should be advised for Ms V for the future?

B2 **Q1**

You are the obstetrics registrar, called to see Mrs Joan Grey in the labour ward. The midwife on duty tells you over the phone: "Mrs Grey has been pushing for two hours, and is getting tired. Please come and assess her."

Q2

What are the conditions that must be satisfied for you to safely perform a forceps delivery?

Q3

What are the potential complications of a forceps delivery?

B3 You are seeing Ms T, who presents with irregular menstrual periods 6 to 12 weeks apart, and excessive hair growth. Please assess her and manage her problem.

Q1

Please take a history of the presenting complaint from Ms T.

Q2

Please ask for relevant examination findings.

Q3

Are there any tests that you would order?

Q4
What are the treatment options for this woman?

B4 Q1
Mrs Ward has presented to the labour ward at 39 weeks gestation with a history of fluid loss from the vagina.

Please assess and advise on management.

The examiner will play the role of the patient.

Q2
Mrs Ward goes home to await the onset of normal labour and agrees to your management plan. She returns the next day with a yellow-green colour to her liquor. Please advise on your management.

Q3
Another woman is on the ward with ruptured membranes at 30 weeks gestation. What features would suggest chorioamnionitis?

B5 Q1
A 49-year-old woman, Mrs Broadbent, presents to you with an 8-week history of increasing abdominal girth, urinary frequency and a palpable abdominal mass.

Please take a history from the patient.

Q2
Please ask for relevant examination findings.

Q3
What investigations would you like to order?

Q4
The results of your investigations show:
- FBE, U+E+Cr, LFTs: normal
- CA125: 1205 U/mL (<45 U/mL)
- CA15.3: 11 U/mL (<30 U/mL)
- CA19.9: 45 U/mL (<39 U/mL)
- CEA 6.4 µg/L (non-smokers <3.5; smokers < 6.5 µg/L)
- LDH 225 U/L (100-230)
- CXR: small pleural effusion in R lung field
- Pelvic ultrasound: Bilateral solid and cystic ovarian masses with low resistance blood flow. Small uterus, endometrial thickness 3 mm, ascites, normal kidneys
- CT scan: Large solid, cystic mass arising from pelvis, ascites, omental thickening, no lymphadenopathy

"Doctor, what do my results show, and what do we do now?"

B6 **Q1**

You are in antenatal clinic. Susan Thompson is a 30-year-old primigravida at 38 weeks gestation. You have just examined her and noted her BP to be 160/100 with a FWT 2+ protein.

"Is there something wrong, doctor?"

Q2

"What happens now, doctor?"

Please advise on management of this patient.

B7 **Q1**

Mrs V presents with hot flushes and night sweats. She has not had a period for 12 months. Please manage her problem.

Q2

Please advise Mrs V on the use of hormone therapy (HT).

Q3

Please advise Mrs V on the benefits and risks of using hormone therapy.

B8 **Q1**

Mrs Tran has been referred to you by her GP with the following letter:

Dear Dr,
I am referring Mrs Tran to you, who is 10 weeks pregnant with recent onset of jaundice. Please manage her pregnancy.
Regards
Dr LMO

You are the doctor. The examiner is playing the role of Mrs Tran.

Q2

Results show:
- Blood group A+, no antibodies
- FBE Hb 130 WCC 6.0 Plts 200
- Rubella immune, TPHA negative, MSU negative, HIV negative, declines Down syndrome screening test
- LFT: AST 250, ALT 500, ALP 50, bilirubin 180, albumin 35
- Hep A negative
- Hep B +ve (HBcAg +ve, anti-HBcIgM +ve, HBsAg +ve, anti-HBsIg −ve, HBe Ag −ve)
- Hep C negative
- Upper abdominal ultrasound: no gallstones detected

Please explain to Mrs Tran how her diagnosis alters your management of her pregnancy.

STUDENT OSCE C

C1 **Q1**

Mrs Gore is a 27-year-old woman presenting to your clinic with a monochorionic diamniotic twin pregnancy. Counsel her as to the increased risks compared with a singleton pregnancy.

Q2

"I have been reading in the paper over the weekend about twin–twin transfusion syndrome. How will we tell if I am developing this condition?"

Q3

Mrs Gore does not develop twin–twin transfusion syndrome during her pregnancy. What conditions and preparations would need to be in place for you to be happy to deliver Mrs Gore's twins vaginally, rather than by caesarean section?

C2 **Q1**

You are the casualty medical officer seeing Mrs Rachel Turner, a 24-year-old primigravida, at roughly 9 weeks gestation, in the Emergency Department. She has presented with PV bleeding. Take a history, examine and initiate investigation of the patient.

Q2

What are the differential diagnoses of the cause of the PV bleeding?

Q3

- Ultrasound report: 6/40 sized intra-uterine gestational sac. No fetal pole or fetal heart visible. Cervical os open
- βHCG = 8000 IU/mL
- Haemoglobin 130 g/dl

What is your management?

Q4

"Tell me what went wrong, doctor." Counsel the patient.

C3 **Q1**

You are called to the labour ward to see Mr and Mrs Harlow, who presented in their first pregnancy at 38 weeks gestation with a 3-day history of reduced fetal movements. They have had a fetal death in utero confirmed on ultrasound, and are understandably distraught.
Take a focused history and advise on appropriate investigations.

Q2

Advise and counsel the couple on subsequent management.

C4 Q1

Ms B presents for an abortion. She is 10 weeks pregnant based on an ultrasound. Please take an appropriate history.

Q2

Please inform Ms B on the process of pregnancy termination and the risks involved.

Q3

What should be advised for Ms B for the future?

C5 Q1

You are attending the delivery of a term infant in the labour ward. At delivery the baby has two loops of cord wrapped tightly around the neck. The baby is blue in colour and not breathing at birth. The liquor was clear at delivery.

Please demonstrate how you would manage the resuscitation of the baby on the doll provided. Explain to the examiner as you go what steps you are taking.

Q2

Explain to the examiner how you would determine the Apgar score for an infant 5 minutes after birth, and why the Apgar score is performed.

C6 Q1

Ms B presents to have a routine Pap smear performed. She last had a normal smear 3 years ago and her smears have always been normal.

Please explain why Pap smears are performed and how often they should be done.

Q2

Please perform a Pap smear on the mannequin. Describe the steps of performing the Pap smear and explain what you are doing to the examiner.

C7 Q1

You are in an antenatal clinic. Mrs Joanne Thompson, a 30-year-old primigravida at 34 weeks gestation is enquiring about pain relief options in labour.

"Hello, doctor. I am a bit worried about how I will cope in labour. What can I do for pain relief?"

Q2

"Can you tell me any advantages or disadvantages between the various options?"

C8 **Encounter 1**
Mrs W, a 62-year-old woman, comes to see you for some advice regarding her family history of cancer.

Please take an appropriate history from Mrs W.

Encounter 2
What advice would you give Mrs W regarding her family history?

Encounter 3
What is the likely hereditary cancer syndrome in this family? What are the other main gynaecological family cancer syndromes, and what are the genes that are mutated?

Encounter 4
What screening tests, and what prophylactic surgery, are available for:
a HNPCC?
b BRCA 1/2?

STUDENT OSCE D

D1 Annabelle Gordon is a 35-year-old primigravida at 34 weeks gestation, who presents via ambulance with an antepartum haemorrhage at 0100 hours. The bleeding is fresh and at least 2 cups in volume, with ongoing bleeding continuing. She has been a regular attendee at antenatal care, with an uneventful pregnancy to date. The 20-week scan showed an anterior, not low placenta. You are attending her.

Please take any further relevant history and say what examination you would conduct, as well as management, based on the history above and your findings.

The examiner will play the role of the patient.

Q1
Please take a brief and directed history.

Q2
Please tell the examiner what physical examination findings you would like to know.

Q3
Please indicate your initial management steps.

Q4
What is your provisional diagnosis?

D2 **Encounter 1**
Mrs D, a 62-year-old woman, is referred to you with the sensation of a lump in her vagina, as well as urinary incontinence.

Please take an appropriate history.

Encounter 2
Please ask for relevant examination findings.

Encounter 3
Please explain to Mrs D what investigations you would like to perform, and what management options are available to her. Outline any relevant health issues you have identified.

D3 **Q1**

You are the obstetrics resident, called to see Mrs Walker, a 25-year-old primigravida, in labour. Please take an appropriate history, examine the patient, and advise on your management.

Q2

The midwife calls you 2 hours later to say that she has heard a deceleration during the last contraction, and that she has put on a CTG monitor. She asks you to come and review the fetal heart trace. What are the features of the trace that you would look for? What features indicate a reassuring CTG?

Q3

Mrs Walker is reassessed by vaginal examination 4 hours after your initial examination, and is found to have a cervical dilatation of 5 cm. Outline your assessment and management.

D4 **Q1**

Ms C, a 24-year-old woman, presents requesting a script for the combined oral contraceptive pill. Please counsel her.

Q2

Please inform Ms C on how to start the COCP and the side effects.

Q3

Please advise Ms C on the benefits and risks of using the COCP.

D5 **Q1**

Mrs Drake is 40 years old, and presents at 9 weeks gestation in her third pregnancy. She wishes to discuss the risk of Down syndrome. Please take a brief history and counsel her.

Q2

"Will an ultrasound pick up Down syndrome, doctor? I would not want to have a Down syndrome child."

Q3

Mrs Drake has a high-risk screening test for Down syndrome (1 in 40). Explain this to her and counsel appropriately.

"What do I need to do now, doctor?"

D6 **Q1**

A 20-year-old woman, Anna, presents for her first Pap smear. She has had an episode of post-coital bleeding in the last week.

Please take a history of the presenting complaint from Anna.

Q2

What investigations would you like to perform at the time of your examination?

Q3

The results of your investigations are:
- Pap smear: normal
- Colposcopy: normal
- HVS:
    - Wet prep – trichomonas absent
    - Gram stain – leukocytes ++, normal vaginal flora
    - Culture – heavy growth of normal vaginal flora
- Chlamydia DNA – positive
- Gonorrhoea DNA – negative

What is your management now?

D7 **Q1**

Mrs Hassim is a 28-year-old recent migrant from Afghanistan presenting to the public antenatal clinic at 8 weeks gestation for her first antenatal visit. She is fully veiled.

Please advise her on the antenatal tests required, and explain to her in lay terms what the tests are for.

Q2

You are seeing her two weeks later. The results of the tests include:
- Blood group: AB +ve, no antibodies
- Full blood examination: Hb 120 (110–140), MCV 69 (80–100), WCC 8.0 (4–11), platelets 280 (150–450)
- RPR: negative
- Hepatitis B serology: negative
- Rubella serology: immune
- HIV serology: negative
- MSU: negative
- Vitamin D: 20 (75–250)

Please explain the significance of any abnormal tests, and what, if anything, needs to be done about them.

D8 **Q1**

Mrs Meadows, a 46-year-old woman, presents with heavy, irregular periods.

Please take a history relevant to the presenting complaint.

Q2
Please ask for relevant examination findings.

Q3
What investigations would you like to order?

Q4
The results of your investigations are as follows:
- Pap smear: normal
- Haemoglobin: 9.7 g/dl
- Iron studies: consistent with Fe-deficiency anaemia
- Normal thyroid, renal and liver function
- Pelvic ultrasound:
  - Endometrium 20 mm thick
  - Uterus 10 cm long, 4.8 cm antero-posterior diameter, 6 cm wide
  - Normal uterus, ovaries and tubes
  - Corpus luteum in left ovary
  - No free fluid in pelvis
- Pipelle (if asked for): endometrial hyperplasia without atypia
  - (If pipelle not asked for) "What would you advise next?"
- Hysteroscopy/D+C findings: endometrial hyperplasia without atypia

How would you manage this patient's problem, and what are the side effects of treatment?

4

Medical student OSCE answers and discussion

STUDENT OSCE A

A1 Q1

History

(Only give history if specifically requested)
- Age at diagnosis: 4 – presented in DKA

  ½ mark
- Insulin dosing regime: 3x daily actrapid, nocte protophane

  ½ mark

Compliance
- Sometimes skips doses if busy
- HBA1c average around 10
- Says her diabetes is 'brittle and difficult to control'
- Sees a diabetes specialist once a year and her GP intermittently
- No eye review for more than a year
- No regular podiatry review
- Unaware of any renal disease
- No hospitalisations for diabetes for last 6 years

  Score any 4
  4 marks

Gynecological history
- Regular cycles 5/28
- No problems with menorrhagia, dysmenorrhoea, dyspareunia
- Last Pap smear – possibly more than 2 years ago
- Regular coitus

  2 marks

Surgical history
- Nil
- Medications: insulin as above, nil else

  ½ mark
- Allergies: penicillin – rash

  ½ mark

Social history
- Schoolteacher
- Married 2 years

• Stable home life and finances

Any 2 scores 1 mark

• Cigarettes/alcohol, recreational or illicit drugs
  – Non-smoker
  – Alcohol × 2 glasses wine per week
  – No recreational drugs

1 mark

Q2
Pre-pregnancy
• Importance of diabetes control: fetal abnormalities and later pregnancy complications related to HbA1c level
• Should not get pregnant until glucose control optimal
• Needs preconceptual diabetitian visit
• Prevention of spina bifida: needs 5 mg of folate rather than 0.5 mg
• Team management required: physician, diabetes educator
• Ancillary services: referral for podiatry, ophthalmology
• Baseline investigations
• Diabetes: HbA1c, 24-hour urine collection, screen for thyroid disease
• Pregnancy: rubella serology

5 marks (any 5 score 1 mark each)

Antenatal management
• Specialist/obstetric unit experienced in management of diabetes
• Experienced ultrasound required
• Tight glucose control required compared to non-pregnant state
• More frequent review compared to general population
• Need for fetal surveillance

3 marks (any 3 score 1 point each)

Labour and delivery
• Timing and mode of delivery will depend upon fetal assessment
• Keep glucose control optimal during labour too
• Vaginal delivery is possible, risk of shoulder dystocia

1 mark

Postnatal care
• Baby to the nursery

1 mark

20 marks total

Discussion
Diabetes affects 7.5% of the Australian adult population. Type I diabetes accounts for 10–15% of diabetes cases, with the rest being type II. These pregnancies are considered high risk due to the potential for complications for the mother and the fetus. A thorough knowledge of the risks (outlined in the ideal answers above) is expected, given the common nature of the condition.

A2 Q1
History
N.B. Should be brief (an obstetric emergency)
- 32-year-old primigravida with a singleton pregnancy
- No other medical or antepartum problems
- Induction of labour 16 hours ago with ARM and IV Syntocinon at 40 weeks gestation
- Contracting 4:10 strong for last 6 hours. Adequate progress on serial VEs
- Liquor clear. CTG normal (apart from no reactivity) throughout labour
- Used 1 dose of pethidine 100 mg 2 hours ago
- Normal cephalic delivery. No episiotomy cut. Duration of second stage 90 minutes
- A baby boy, with 1 and 5 minute Apgars of 8 and 9
  ½–1½ marks, depending on degree of detail about labour obtained
- Placenta appears whole. Third stage lasted 10 minutes
  ½ mark
- Bleeding heavily after delivery of placenta, fresh blood plus clots. Estimated blood loss 1 L
  ½ mark
- Medications: Syntocinon (10 units in 1 L N/saline, running at 120 mL/hour)

Examination/management
(Obstetric emergency, so carry on at same time)
- Call for more help (extra midwife/midwives, other doctors if available)
  ½ mark
- Assess patient's conscious state – patient drowsy, but conscious and orientated

Assess haemodynamic state
- BP 100/60, PR 100, still active fresh bleeding, peripheries cool and sweaty
  ½ mark

Initiate resuscitation
- 2 wide bore (16 gauge) IV lines
  – Send off blood for group and cross-match, FBE, clotting profile (APTT/INR/DIC screen), Haemacue (if available)
  – Bed to be moved into head-down position
  – Give O_2 by mask, and use O_2 saturation monitor if available
  – Give colloid agent IV (Gelafusion)
  – Cross-match 4 units of blood, but use O negative blood if necessary
  – Observations every 10–15 minutes by midwife to be recorded
  ½–1 mark depending on completeness of resuscitation Mx

Establish the cause of the PPH

1 Uterine atony (most likely)
  Abdominal Ex shows 'boggy', non-contracted, enlarged uterus with
  fundus above the umbilicus

  1 mark

2 Retained placenta/products
  Placenta and membranes complete; no expulsion of further products
  on application of fundal pressure

  1 mark

3 Vaginal/perineal lacerations
  No vaginal lacerations on Sims speculum Ex

  ½ mark

4 Cervical laceration
  No cervical lacerations with careful 'walking' around the cervical
  circumference with sponge forceps during speculum Ex

  ½ mark

5 Haemostatic disorders
  • Await results of clotting profile

Medical management of uterine atony

*N.B. Continue to prompt candidate to run through further stages of
management if necessary, by pointing out that the patient is continuing to
bleed/deteriorate.*

• Bimanual uterine fundal massage

  ½ mark

• 10 unit bolus of Syntocinon to be given IV
• 40 units of Syntocinon into 1 L of Hartmanns, running over 4 hours

  1 mark, ½ without correct dose

• Ergometrine 500 mcg, with half IV and half IM

  1 mark, ½ without correct dose

• Insert indwelling urinary catheter

  1 mark

• Misoprostol tablets (200 mcg per tablet), 2–4 tablets per vagina/rectum

"The patient is still bleeding – now a total of 2.5 litres according to the
midwives."

Surgical management of uterine atony

• Call for help (experienced obstetrician if available), and take to
  operating theatre
• General anaesthetic (consider central venous line with anaesthetist)
• Examine in theatre: no lacerations or retained products, but continued
  bleeding
• Give prostaglandin F2α (0.25 mg injected via abdomen, by steadying
  fundus with non-injecting hand, into 4 quadrants of the uterus:
  maximum dose 1 mg)

  1 mark, ½ without correct dose

Move to laparotomy (midline)
- Uterine artery ligation bilaterally
- Internal iliac artery ligation (bilateral)
- Consider B-Lynch suture
- Uterine packing or intrauterine tamponade balloon may be considered
  ½ mark for any of the above 4 options, to maximum 1½ marks
- If all else fails – hysterectomy (total or subtotal)
  ½ mark

N.B. An experienced obstetrician is able to attend. A hysterectomy, while considered, is not necessary to control the patient's bleeding.
14 marks total for Q1

Q2
- Past history of post-partum haemorrhage
- Prolonged labour
- Precipitate labour
- Prolonged use of IV syntocinon
- Ante-partum haemorrhage/abruption ('Couvelaire uterus')
- Grand-multiparity (reduced uterine tone)
- Uterine overdistension (multiple pregnancy, polyhydramnios, fetal macrosomia)
- Instrumental/operative delivery
- Uterine fibroids
- Chorioamnionitis
- Uterine trauma (rupture/inversion)
- Disorders of haemostasis (inherited – Von Willebrands, haemophilia carriers; acquired – thrombocytopaenias, disseminated intravascular coagulation)
  ½ mark for each mentioned risk factor to maximum of 3 marks

Q3
In the next labour the patient is at increased risk of postpartum haemorrhage, and should be managed as a high-risk patient.
1 mark

Precautions include:
- IV access in next labour *(½ mark)*
- Send off FBE and group and hold at start of labour *(½ mark)*
- Experienced accoucher to be present at the delivery *(½ mark)*
- Ergometrine and misoprostol to be readily available *(½ mark)*
- Ensure delivery suite has prostaglandin F2α in stock
  3 marks total for Q3

Discussion
Post-partum haemorrhage (PPH) is defined as the loss of greater then 500 mL of blood after delivery. It can be divided into *primary* (within

24 hours of delivery) and *secondary* (fresh bleeding after 24 hours but before 6 weeks post-delivery), which have different differential causes. The causes of secondary PPH include retained products (placenta or membranes), infection (chorioamnionitis/endometritis), subinvolution of the placental site, and rare causes such as aretrio-venous malformations. Our discussion will be limited to primary PPH, presented in this OSCE case.

Worldwide, PPH remains a major cause of maternal mortality and morbidity. The Western world has experienced a significant decline in maternal deaths from PPH due to preventative management (i.e. expectant management of the third stage of labour), as well as the ready availability of blood transfusions and oxytocic therapy. Nonetheless, deaths, as well as serious morbidity, due to post-partum haemorrhage still occur in Australia. In Victoria, for the years 1997–2003, there were 13 direct maternal deaths, of which five (38%) were attributed to PPH (two from amniotic fluid embolus and subsequent DIC, one from abruption causing uterine atony, one from uterine fibroids, and one from a retained placenta).

The incidence of primary PPH is estimated to be around 5% in most Australian obstetric units. It is a common obstetric complication, with potentially very serious consequences and, as such, students would be expected to complete their obstetrics rotation with a clear approach to management, and do well on this OSCE station.

The most common cause of primary PPH is uterine atony. The next two most common causes are retained products of conception and genital tract laceration (of the vagina or cervix). A rare cause of PPH is coagulopathy. A list of the risk factors for PPH are found in the answer to Q2.

The management of primary PPH is clearly laid out in the worked answer. It is important in this OSCE to state the obvious steps that would be taken in such an obstetric emergency, such as calling for help and giving oxygen by mask. If you do not say that you would take those steps the examiner cannot assume that you would automatically take them! In real life, as a resident or registrar in a tertiary hospital, there are well-trained staff who would do this automatically, but in the exam situation you are on your own and must demonstrate that you know how to handle an emergency.

A key approach to answering the management of a PPH is to divide it into clear sections, as laid out in the examiner's ideal answer:
1 Call for help.
2 Initial assessment.
3 Initiate resuscitation.
4 Establish the most likely cause of PPH on history, examination and investigation.
5 Specific treatment of the cause of PPH.

If cause of PPH is vaginal/cervical laceration, then obviously suturing of the laceration should control the bleeding, and may need to be done in theatre (allows for both better visualisation, trained theatre nurse for assistance, and expert anaesthetic staff for ongoing resuscitation effort while bleeding brought under control).

If the PPH is due to a retained placenta or products, then a manual removal of placental tissue under adequate analgesia is required. In this case, premature administration of oxytocics may cause the cervix to clamp shut and make the procedure much more difficult. Conversely, a general anaesthetic may relax the uterine muscle, making it easier for the uterus to admit the hand for separation of the placenta from its attachment to the uterine wall.

Any identified coagulopathy should be corrected. Thrombocytopaenias will be corrected with platelet transfusion, while disseminated intravascular coagulation (DIC) will be corrected with fresh frozen plasma/cryoprecipitate and platelets. With coagulopathies, a haematologist (if available) should be consulted to help guide the appropriate administration of blood products.

Remember that the uterine atony is overwhelmingly the most common cause of primary PPH. It is the first, second and third cause on any list, to emphasise its importance. Management should start with medical treatment, and students are expected to know correct dosages. In an emergency there will often not be time to look up doses, so they must be memorised. Some of the potential side effects of the various oxytocics (not mentioned in the ideal answer as they do not relate to the presented case) are:

- Syntocinon – hypotension (especially as a large IV bolus), hyponatremia (due to antidiuretic effect), can cause ECG changes with IV boluses
- Ergometrine – nausea and vomiting, hypertension
- Misoprostol – bronchoconstriction (beware with asthma sufferers), fever, nausea
- Prostaglandin F2α – bronchoconstriction, nausea, vomiting, diarrhoea, fever, hypertension

All of the above oxytocics can cause cramping uterine pains as the uterus contracts.

Severe PPH can result in hypovolaemic shock, DIC and (rarely) Sheehan's syndrome. Sheehan's syndrome is avascular necrosis of the pituitary secondary to severe obstetric haemorrhage, and occurs in 1 in 10,000 deliveries. The patient has subsequent deficiency of the anterior pituitary hormones, manifested as failed lactation, amenorrhoea, hypothyroidism, and adrenocorticoid deficiency.

Primary prevention of PPH is extremely important to reduce the incidence of this obstetric complication. 'Active management' of the third stage of labour reduces the risk of PPH by 40%. It includes the administration of an oxytocic agent (usually Syntocinon 10 IU) prophylactically at delivery, after the delivery of the anterior shoulder of the baby, as well as early cord clamping (hastens placental separation), and delivery of the placenta with controlled cord traction. Retained placenta is a major cause of PPH, and if retained longer than 30 minutes, a manual removal should be performed. The Brandt-Andrews method (controlled cord traction with suprapubic pressure on the uterus to prevent uterine inversion, after positive signs of placental separation have been witnessed) helps to reduce the time to delivery of the placenta.

Secondary prevention is where a patient has experienced a PPH in a previous delivery. Care should be taken to optimise haemoglobin with haematinics prior to the onset of labour. The other key points are listed in the answers to Q3.

A3 Q1

- Vital signs to be checked on ward: (pulse rate, respiratory rate, blood pressure, oxygen saturation, temperature)
  - Every 15 minutes for first hour
  - Every 30 minutes for the next 3 hours
  - Every hour for the following 6 hours
  - 4-hourly thereafter

1 mark

- Urine output to be measured hourly: notify if <30 mL per hour
- Start a strict fluid balance chart

1 mark

- Administer intravenous fluids
  - 1 L normal saline at 8/24ly rate (125 mL/hour), followed by
  - 1 L normal saline at 8/24ly rate, followed by
  - 5% dextrose at 8/24ly rate

1 mark

- DVT (deep venous thrombosis) prophylaxis
  - Low molecular weight or sodium heparin
  - Graduated compression stockings
  - +/– intermittent pneumatic compression

2 marks

- Analgesia
  - PCA
  - Paracetamol 1 g 6/24ly either PR or IV

1 mark

- Nil by mouth (ice chips for comfort)

1 mark

- Antibiotics – not indicated unless evidence of infection (prophylactic antibiotics given at time of operation)
- Blood tests to be performed the next morning:
  - FBE
  - Urea, electrolytes, creatinine
  - Albumin (may lose large amounts in malignant ascites)

1 mark

Q2
History
- Well until this morning
- Vomited twice
- Generalised abdominal pain and distension
- Burping frequently

- Has not passed flatus

2 marks

Examination
- BP 120/80, PR 90 bpm, afebrile, O_2 saturation 96% on room air, RR 16
- Urine output 35 mL/hour
- Cardiovascular/respiratory Ex:
  - JVP +1
  - Dual heart sounds, nil added sounds
  - Dull to percussion at lung bases; no crepitations
- Abdominal Ex:
  - Distended abdomen
  - Wound clean and dry
  - No bowel sounds to auscultation

4 marks

Q3
- Chest X-ray
- Abdominal X-ray (supine and erect)
- FBE, urea + electrolytes, creatinine

3 marks

Q4
- Diagnosis: post-operative bowel ileus

Management
- IV fluids
- Naso-gastric tube if vomiting persists
- Antiemetics
- Review analgesia (if can reduce opioids by using NSAIDs, may benefit bowel function)
- Nil by mouth until bowel sounds present/passing flatus

3 marks
20 marks total

Discussion
This scenario tests the ability of the student to manage a patient having a major abdominal procedure in the immediate post-operative period. The second part of the station requires the student to recognise and manage a common post-operative problem (post-operative bowel ileus).

A4 Q1

Mr and Mrs F have been married for 5 years and Mrs F ceased using the combined oral contraceptive pill 3 years ago in order to become pregnant. She is 37 years old and has never been pregnant in the past.

She has 28–30-day cycles and the periods last 4 days. She has never had a problem with her periods.

- No past history of STDs/PID
- Last Pap smear was 3 years ago
- Mr F is 40 years old and has never fathered any children
- No past history of surgery or injury to testes, or of mumps orchitis
- They are both healthy with no other personal history of note
- They have sex 2–3 times a week
- They have no family history of note
- They are non-smokers and occasionally drink alcohol. She is taking folic acid supplementation at a dose of 1 mg/day
- She is a primary school teacher and he is a secondary school teacher
- They are both very frustrated about their inability to become pregnant

8 marks total (depending on completeness of history)

Q2
Relevant examination findings for Mrs F are:
- Normal BP and BMI 22
- Vaginal examination shows a normal size anteverted uterus which is mobile and non-tender and there are no masses palpable. A Pap smear is performed. If other examination asked for, it is normal.

4 marks total

Relevant examination findings for Mr F:
- Mr F has a normal pattern of body hair and a male habitus. BMI is 24
- He has 15 mL testicles bilaterally. There are no other findings.

3 marks total

(NB: Common error is to forget to examine the male partner)

Q3
- Female hormonal profile including testing for ovarian reserve (days 2–4 FSH, LH, E_2), mid luteal progesterone and TSH

2 marks

- Rubella and varicella immunity

1 mark

- Testing of tubal patency with laparoscopy, hysteroscopy, dye studies, D&C or hysterosalpingogram

1 mark

- SA and IBT (semen analysis and immunobead test for anti-sperm antibodies)

1 mark

20 marks total

Discussion
The definition of infertility is one year of unprotected intercourse without conception. Fifteen per cent of couples are infertile (sterile and subfertile); 3 per cent of couples are sterile due to azospermia, absent ovulation or female genital tract obstruction. One in 7 couples are infertile at age 30–34 years, 1 in 5 at age 35–39 years and 1 in 4 at age 40–44 years.

Infertility is a growing problem and may be due to a number of factors: 1) postponement of childbearing; 2) increasing and effective use of contraception; 3) greater accessibility to abortion; 4) rising incidence of sexually transmitted infections (STI), especially in developing countries; and 5) possible environmental toxins. Smokers take longer to become pregnant and are also at greater risk of spontaneous abortion.

In each ovulatory cycle a couple has a 20–25% chance of pregnancy (monthly probability of conception or fecundability). After 3 months of exposure 65% of couples are pregnant, after 6 months 75% are pregnant, after 1 year 85% are pregnant and after 2 years 95% are pregnant. Most infertility investigations are carried out after one year of infertility, except in a woman over the age of 35 years, when investigation should be begun after 6 months of infertility.

Infertility is classified as primary (never pregnant) or secondary (has been pregnant, no matter the outcome).

It is important that a history and examination are performed on the couple. Key points to note from each are their age, the duration of the infertility and whether it is primary or secondary, and if pregnancies have occurred outside the current partnership. A sexual history should be obtained taking note of the frequency of sexual intercourse and whether it is timed to ovulation.

For the woman the history should involve the frequency of the menstrual cycle, its duration and other associated factors such as heavy bleeding or pain. Prior obstetric and gynaecological history, such as the occurrence of an STI, as well as medical and surgical history and family history, are important. There are some medical conditions, such as pulmonary artery hypertension, that preclude pregnancy. The use of medications (prescribed and over-the-counter), as well as the use of cigarettes, alcohol and illicit drugs should be noted. A general and gynaecological examination should be performed, taking note of the size of the uterus, its position, shape and mobility, as well as the size of the ovaries, if able to be palpated. Tenderness on examination should be noted. A Pap smear must be done if due.

For the man the past and current history is important, such as the occurrence of an STI or a mumps infection as an adult. Prior surgical history is also important to note, such as an orchidopexy. The use of medications (prescribed and over-the-counter), as well as the use of cigarettes, alcohol and illicit drugs, should be noted. A general and scrotal examination should be performed, taking note of the size, shape and consistency of the testes, as well as the presence of the vas deferens, varicocoele, hydrocoele or hernia.

The **aetiology** of infertility is varied and often more than one problem may be present in each couple. The following are possible causes of infertility:
- Male
- Ovulatory
- Tubal
- Age

- Endometriosis
- Coital
- Cervical and uterine
- Unexplained.

The more severe the diagnosed cause of infertility, the better the prognosis for conception after treatment, provided that the treatment completely corrects the problem. Minor abnormalities alone may not have an impact, but when they occur in combination the probability of pregnancy may be very low. The duration of infertility and the time remaining for conception may be more important than the cause of infertility itself.

Male infertility

Most causes of male infertility are not amenable to treatment. The most common problem is a decrease in sperm production (*hypospermatogenesis*) as a result of a testicular problem. This may be acquired as a result of mumps infection or it may be congenital as a result of a chromosomal problem such as Klinefelter's syndrome. Six per cent of men with severe oligospermia (concentration $<10 \times 10^6$/mL) have a karyotypic abnormality and some of these men may also have a genetic problem with sperm production which involves a deletion of a part of their Y chromosome that is important in sperm production.

Males may also have an obstructive cause for their infertility. This may be acquired due to epididymo-orchitis secondary to an STI or as a result of vasectomy, or it could be congenital, such as due to congenital absence of the vas deferens. In most obstructive causes the male presents with azospermia.

Rarely, hypospermatogenesis may be due to a hypothalamic problem such as congenital Kallman's syndrome or a pituitary problem such as a prolactinoma. In these cases there is a lack of stimulation of the testis by FSH and LH. These causes are amenable to treatment.

The testes also produce testosterone and some men with severe male infertility may need to consider testosterone replacement therapy once their infertility treatment is completed.

Ovulatory disorders

The most common disorder of ovulation that affects fertility is polycystic ovarian syndrome (PCOS). Women with this disorder have oligo-ovulation and are often hirsute and obese.

Other causes for ovulatory infertility may be due to hypothalamic problems such as weight loss or a pituitary disorder such as prolactinoma. In these cases there is no stimulation of the ovary because of a disorder of production of FSH and LH.

The ovary may not be responsive to stimulation. This is termed premature ovarian failure and is not amenable to infertility therapy.

Tubal factor

Tubal factor infertility is secondary to pelvic inflammatory disease (PID). The increasing incidence of STIs, which cause PID and tubal damage, is responsible for the increasing incidence of infertility, particularly in developing countries. The most common organisms that cause PID are *Chlamydia trachomatis* and *Neisseria gonorrhoea*. The problem with both these STIs is that they are often asymptomatic at the time of infection and therefore go untreated; a tubal factor is diagnosed later at the time of infertility investigation when pelvic adhesions and tubal damage are found, such as a hydrosalpinx. Other causes for tubal and pelvic disease are related to the presence of pelvic adhesions due to previous surgery (e.g. ruptured appendix), as well as inflammatory bowel disease (e.g. Crohn's disease).

Age
There is a definite age-related decline in fertility. In a study of women in a donor insemination program it was shown that there is a progressive decline in the pregnancy rate after the age of 30 years. One-third of women who defer pregnancy until over the age of 35 years will have an infertility problem. For the 40–44-year-old age group the monthly fecundity rate is about 5%, while it is negligible in women 45–49 years old, when only 2–5% will have a viable pregnancy.

Age-related decline in infertility is due to the quantity and quality of oocytes still present, as well as the greater likelihood of the presence of conditions such as endometriosis. There is also a greater likelihood for spontaneous abortion in older women, reaching a rate of almost 50% in a woman older than 40 years. This is mostly due to autosomal trisomies.

Endometriosis
Endometriosis is the presence of ectopic endometrial tissue in the pelvis. With every menstrual cycle this tissue bleeds and is irritating to the peritoneum. It is the reason for the dysmenorrhoea that is experienced by women with this disease. The areas heal by scarring and can therefore cause adhesions and a distortion of the pelvic anatomy. This distortion is the most likely reason for the infertility experienced by women with endometriosis.

Coital problems
These problems may be related to either physical (diabetes, alcohol, medications – e.g. anti-androgens, antihypertensives) and/or psychological causes of impotence in the male. There may also be an inability to ejaculate into the vagina due to hypospadius. Female problems include psychological factors causing vaginismus as well as physical factors related to problems in the vagina such as occur after radiotherapy.

Cervical and uterine factors
The only definite and rare reasons for cervical factor infertility are due to conisation of the cervix by whatever method and cervical amputation (Manchester repair). These procedures may cause cervical stenosis and lack of mucus production. The cervix and cervical mucus are important because they: 1) aid sperm receptivity; 2) protect the sperm from the hostile acidic and phagocytic vaginal environment; 3) supplement energy for sperm metabolism; 4) filter abnormal and nonmotile sperm; and 5) act as a sperm reservoir. Also the cervix is a possible site for sperm capacitation.

Uterine factors include uterine adhesions, which are often acquired as a result of surgery or infection. Uterine leiomyomas and polyps as a cause of infertility remains controversial. In general, these factors are more likely related to abortion rather than infertility.

Unexplained infertility

Couples with idiopathic infertility may have subtle ovulatory, tubal and/or sperm functional problems that are unable to be diagnosed by current technology. Couples with idiopathic infertility have a 35–50% cumulative pregnancy rate after 2 years of follow-up and 60–70% rate after 3 years of follow-up. However, if they are infertile for 4 or more years they have a very poor prognosis. The rate of spontaneous pregnancies in these couples also decreases with age of the female partner.

It is mandatory that both partners be investigated. **Investigations** are those that will alter the management plan. The basic infertility investigations include: 1) semen analysis and sperm antibody assessment (SA+IBT); 2) tubal assessment; 3) hormonal assessment, including tests of ovarian reserve and ovulation and thyroid function. Rubella and varicella immunity should also be performed and the female immunised if she is not immune. Other hormonal tests will need to be considered if an ovulatory disorder is suspected.

Semen analysis and sperm antibody assessment is based on strict World Health Organization (WHO) criteria. A normal SA is a:

- volume of 2–5 mL
- pH 7.2–7.8
- concentration of greater than 20×10^6/mL
- greater than 50% motility, further defined depending on the type of movement and its speed
- greater than 15% normal forms
- less than 1×10^6/mL WBC.

The viscosity of the semen is noted and liquefaction should take place within 30 min. Fructose content (seminal vesicle) and acid phosphatase (prostate) can also be assessed. The period of abstinence prior to a semen analysis should be 2–3 days and the specimen should be collected by masturbation. If not performed in the office, it should be examined within 1 h of production. If 1 SA is abnormal it should be repeated at least twice, one month apart, for a male factor problem to be diagnosed.

Sperm antibodies should be assessed routinely as 6% of men have these antibodies for no apparent reason. The antibodies can be localised to the head, midpiece or tail and can affect sperm movement or fertilisation by preventing the sperm from recognising the egg. About 50% of men who have had a vasectomy reversal develop sperm antibodies and about 50% of such men father children.

The most comprehensive **assessment of the pelvis**, tubal normality and patency and endometrial normality is performed with a laparoscopy and hysteroscopy. A hysterosalpingogram (HSG) can also be performed, although it only gives information on tubal patency and normality. It is best considered if a woman has a contraindication or is at high risk of complication at laparoscopic surgery. Both tests for tubal patency may be therapeutic.

All women should be assessed for **ovarian reserve**. At Monash IVF, an FSH greater than 10 IU/L and an E_2 greater than 200 pmol/mL is considered abnormal and guarded prognosis given to the woman in terms of treatment success. An FSH greater than 20 IU/L is an indication for the use of donor oocytes. A high E_2 (>200 pmol/mL) with a normal FSH may indicate earlier follicular recruitment which will mask an otherwise high FSH and also indicates a poor prognosis. A basal FSH concentration may be a better predictor of fertility outcome than age. Women who smoke have a higher FSH level as do women with one ovary. A **mid luteal progesterone concentration (MLP)** can also be useful. A serum P concentration less than 5 nmol/mL is diagnostic of anovulation if performed at the correct time. The ideal concentration on day 21 of a 28-day cycle should be greater than 30 nmol/mL. With differing cycle lengths the time that the MLP is assessed will change.

Thyroid assessment, such as a TSH, should be routinely performed in all women with infertility. Hypothyroidism in particular is often silent and can contribute to infertility, particularly by affecting the menstrual cycle. It is easily treated. Hypothyroidism in the mother can cause hypothyroidism in the fetus, which can cause slow brain development.

The **treatment** of the couple is geared towards the cause for their infertility and the number of factors that are present. At all points they should be involved in treatment decisions. If no cause for the infertility is diagnosed this does not mean that there is no treatment and once again they should be allowed to choose what to do, particularly the no-treatment or conservative option.

If a male factor is diagnosed and is amenable to treatment this should be undertaken. However, most males cannot be treated and their infertility is bypassed with the use of in vitro fertilisation (IVF), most often with microinjection (IVF and ICSI), where each of the female's eggs that are retrieved are injected with a motile sperm.

Tubal factor infertility is also often bypassed with the use of IVF. Endometriosis-related infertility can be treated surgically to normalise the anatomy, but can also be treated with IVF if severe.

Ovulatory disorders are often treated medically and if they are the only cause present, successful induction of ovulation will often give the couple the same chance of pregnancy as those where the female ovulates regularly.

The use of 0.4 mg supplemental folic acid is important and should be begun at least 3 months before the couple try for a pregnancy. If not started then they should be begun when they present. This dose has been shown to decrease the risk of neural tube defects.

The three most significant prognostic factors for infertile couples are the period of infertility, female age and the type of infertility. With proper evaluation and treatment at least 50% of couples who attend an infertility clinic will become pregnant. When couples become pregnant there is no difference in obstetric outcome than there is for a fertile couple, taking into account their age, parity and the presence of a multiple pregnancy.

Some couples will never become pregnant with or without treatment and they may choose to remain childless or to adopt. In Australia adoption is difficult because there are few babies offered for adoption. In addition, all adoptions in Victoria are open. International adoption is often easier but can be expensive. In general, adoption is a positive alternative for those who want mostly to be parents. Most adoptions are successful and most adoptees are emotionally healthy and consider it to be a positive experience.

The major shift in the **emotional** aspect of infertility is that emotional stress is viewed as a result of infertility rather than as a cause of infertility. Infertility and its treatment often cause psychological, social, physical and financial stresses on a couple and it has been described as a 'life crisis'. Because infertility is viewed as a medical disease that can be treated, couples often delay crucial decisions about career and life plans, adoption and the possibility of childlessness. For women the experience can be devastating as infertility becomes the focus of their existence and affects nearly all aspects of their lives, including their job security. Women often feel guilty and this guilt may be focused on sexual behaviours as well as feelings of anger and sadness. For men the infertility work-up and treatment may also be stressful as it is seen to be based on performance appraisal and expectation. Sexual dysfunction and impotence may result.

Most infertile couples feel socially isolated as infertility is still viewed as socially unacceptable. The couple will evolve psychologically through a number of phases including surprise, denial, anger, isolation, guilt, grief and finally resolution. They often experience the sense of losing control over their lives.

All couples experiencing infertility would probably benefit from psychological counselling. The most benefit is probably gained at the beginning of the work-up, when a psychiatric indication is present and at the termination of unsuccessful treatment, which represents a crisis for most couples. Group therapy is often beneficial.

References
American Fertility Society Guideline For Practice 1995 Age related infertility.

Bostofte E, Bagger P, Michael A et al 1993 Fertility prognosis for infertile couples. Fertility and Sterility 59:102

Cameron I T, O'Shea F C, Rolland J M et al 1987 Occult ovarian failure: A syndrome of infertility, regular menses and elevated FSH concentrations. Journal of Clinical Endocrinology and Metabolism 67:1190

Cooper G S, Baird D P, Hulka B S et al 1995 Follicle stimulating hormone concentration in relation to active and passive smoking. Obstetrics and Gynecology 85:407

Cramer D W, Barbieri R J, Xu H et al 1994 Determinants of basal follicle-stimulating hormone levels in premenopausal women. Journal of Clinical Endocrinology and Metabolism 79:1105

Edelmann R J, Connolly K J 1986 Psychological aspects of infertility. British Journal of Medical Psychology 59:9

Kennedy S, Robinson J, Hallam N 1993 LLETZ and infertilty. British Journal of Obstetric Gynaecology 100:965

Keye W R 1994 Unexplained infertility. Endocrine and Fertility Forum 15:1

Khalif A E, Toner J P, Muasher S J et al 1992 Significance of basal follicle-stimulating hormone levels in women with one ovary in a program of in vitro fertilization. Fertility and Sterility 57:835

Li T C, Macleod I, Singhal V et al 1991 The obstetric and neonatal outcome of pregnancy in women with a previous history of infertility: a prospective study. British Journal of Obstetric Gynaecology 98:1087

Shalev E, Eliyahu S, Ziv M et al 1994 Routine thyroid function tests in infertile women: are they necessary? American Journal of Obstetric Gynaecology 171:1191

Speroff L, Glass R H, Kase N G 1989 Clinical gynecologic endocrinology and infertility, 4th edn. Williams & Wilkins, Baltimore

Toner J P, Philput C B, Jones G S et al 1991 Basal follicle stimulating hormone level is a better predictor of in vitro fertilization performance than age. Fertility and Sterility 55:784

Van Noord-Zaadstra B M, Looman C W N, Alsbach H et al 1991 Delayed child bearing: effect of age on fecundity and outcome of pregnancy. British Medical Journal 302:1361

Wood C, Calderon I, Crombie A 1992 Age and fertility: Results of assisted reproductive technology in women over 40 years. Journal of Assisted Reproduction and Genetics 9:482

World Health Organization 1999 Laboratory manual for examination of human semen and sperm-cervical mucous interaction, 4th edn. Cambridge University Press, Cambridge, UK

A5   Q1

Smoking and pregnancy

It is extremely important to try to give up smoking prior to attempting to get pregnant, if possible. Smoking has important consequences for fertility and for the pregnancy.

The patient should be referred to QUIT line and encouraged to use therapies to aid smoking cessation, such as nicotine replacement therapy (gum or patches) or hypnotherapy, combined with counselling.

2 marks

As the patient is trying to conceive, she should be encouraged to be on folate supplements to reduce the risk of neural tube defects, have her Pap smears up to date, and her rubella serology checked.

1 mark

The patient needs to be counselled in a non-adversarial manner about the following effects on her reproductive health:

- Smoking increases the risk of infertility (by 54%) and increases delay of conception. This effect is seen with smoking by either partner, and even from exposure to passive smoke
- Smoking causes accelerated ovarian follicle depletion. Menopause occurs 1–4 years earlier in smokers than in non-smokers
- Increased risk of spontaneous miscarriage in smokers
- Increased risk of ectopic pregnancy in smokers (but difficult to control for confounding associated lifestyle factors)
- In IVF, smoking is associated with increased gonadotrophin requirements, reduced estradiol levels, increased number of cancelled cycles, reduced numbers of oocytes collected, reduced fertilisation and implantation rates. It increases failure at every stage of treatment
- It is inadvisable for smokers over the age of 35 to be an estrogen-containing oral contraceptive pill, due to the increased risk of cardio-vascular disease (although not an issue for this woman in the short term)

2 marks for appropriate manner and lay terminology while counselling patient
½ mark for each effect (max 3 marks)

The patient needs to be counselled regarding the risks to her baby from smoking during pregnancy.

Antenatal risks
- Placental abruption
- Premature delivery and premature rupture of membranes
- Placenta praevia
- Lower birth weight (an average of 200 g)

Post-partum risks
- Increased risk of brain tumours in infant
- Increased perinatal mortality rate
- Increased risk of sudden infant death syndrome (SIDS): doubled risk of smoking during pregnancy, tripled if smoking post-natally
- Increased risk of respiratory illness in infants

1 mark for each antenatal/postpartum risk (max 6 marks)

Alcohol and pregnancy
The patient must be advised that there is no safe level of alcohol consumption in pregnancy. Even 'social' drinking cannot be deemed to be safe in pregnancy, and the patient should stop drinking while attempting to conceive and during pregnancy.

1 mark

'Heavy' drinking is associated with:
- fetal alcohol syndrome
- growth restriction
- intellectual impairment and behavioural disturbance
- congenital cardiac, brain and spine defects
- characteristic facial features (low-set ears, small head, hypoplastic philtrum, elongated flat mid-face, short palpebral fissures)

- intellectual impairment, even in the absence of the full fetal alcohol syndrome.

2 marks (1 for each)

Q2
Nicotine replacement therapy contains less nicotine than cigarette smoke, with none of the other toxic substances in cigarettes. Use in pregnancy is safer than smoking, and may improve birthweight if it leads to less smoking.
- Yes, the patient may use nicotine patches or gum to aid smoking cessation in pregnancy.

2 marks

Q3
- Cocaine use in pregnancy is particularly associated with risk of placental abruption.

1 mark

Discussion
The well-documented effects of smoking on cardiovascular disease, cancers and lung disease are not the subject of this OSCE, and have no marks assigned to them. The candidate has been asked to concentrate on reproductive and pregnancy complications.

About 25% of reproductive-age women smoke, with 30% of them quitting or significantly reducing their habit prior to or soon after conceiving a child. The risk of smoking in pregnancy is higher among young women, women from low socio-economic backgrounds, and women who use drugs of abuse. Smoking in pregnancy is a major public health issue, and as such, medical students would be expected to have a thorough knowledge of the risks to a pregnancy. The risks to female reproductive and obstetric health are clearly outlined in the model answer above.

Alcohol use or abuse in pregnancy is inadvisable, due to the outlined risks. While clear evidence of fetal effects has only been demonstrated for 'heavy' alcohol intake, just what 'heavy' intake is defined as is controversial, and there are likely to be more subtle effects on intellectual and behavioural functioning, even with low levels of 'social' alcohol intake in pregnancy.

This is a counselling station, so there is minimal or no history-taking, and the examinee should be directed by the examiner to counsel the patient. The better candidates will provide information in clear layman's terms. Complex medical terminology must be presented in a manner that a non-medical patient can understand.

While the patient has specifically asked about nicotine replacement therapy, another option is the use of bupropion (Zyban). Bupropion is an effective antidepressant, but may also aid in smoking cessation programs. There are no known harmful effects of Zyban in pregnancy, although patients should be encouraged to quit before pregnancy rather than during.

A6 Q1
History
- 70-year-old woman
- Three episodes of bright PV bleeding in last 6 weeks
- Last episode yesterday, with bright red blood and a small blood clot. Still has some dark discharge today
- Menopausal since age 52
- Was on hormone therapy (oestrogen and progestin tablets) for 5–6 years, then stopped age 57
- Has not had a Pap smear in >10 years; never had a mammogram
- Para 3 (all NVDs), 5 grandchildren
- Past medical/surgical Hx:
  - cholecystectomy, appendicectomy, R total knee replacement, tubal ligation
  - type 2 diabetes (on metformin 500 mg BD; BSLs > 8.0 three times/ week)
- NKA
- Non-smoker, occasional wine with dinner
- Family Hx: bowel cancer (father and 1 brother); has colonoscopy every 2 years
- Social Hx: retired teacher, lives with husband, active (gardening and looking after grandchildren)

10 marks, depending on completeness of history

Q2
Examination
- BP 170/95, BMI 35
- Breast Ex: normal
- Chest clear
- Abdominal Ex: obese, large pannus, open cholecystectomy scar, no palpable masses
- Dark blood on pad
- Vulva/vagina: normal appearance
- Speculum: cervix normal; some dark blood coming through the os; Pap smear taken
- Bimanual pelvic Ex: unhelpful due to body habitus

5 marks, depending on completeness

Q3
- FBE, urea + electrolytes, liver function tests
- CXR, ECG
- Transvaginal pelvic ultrasound
- Hysteroscopy/dilatation + curettage
- Mammogram

2 marks

Q4
- Ultrasound features:
  - Endometrial thickness (should be < 4 mm in post-menopausal woman)
  - Morphology of the ovaries
  - Uterine size/dimensions

2 marks

Q5
Surgical staging, including:
- total abdominal hysterectomy
- bilateral salpingo-oophorectomy
- +/– pelvic lymph node sampling

1 mark

20 marks total

Discussion
The patient depicted in this OSCE is at risk for endometrial cancer because of her obesity, her age and her diabetes. In this patient's case, given that the PV bleeding is recurring, a hysteroscopy and curettage would be indicated even with an endometrial lining on ultrasound within normal limits. However, some gynaecologists faced with a patient with a single episode of post-menopausal bleeding would be happy not to proceed with a hysteroscopy, as long as the ultrasound did not show a thickening of the endometrium.

While surgical staging for endometrial cancer has traditionally been performed via a laparotomy, some gynaecological oncologists opt to perform the operation laparoscopically (a total laparoscopic hysterectomy, bilateral salpingo-oophorectomy, and pelvic lymph node dissection). There is currently a trial (LACE) looking at the use of laparoscopic surgery rather than laparotomy for endometrial cancer.

A7 **Q1**
If the candidate starts to take a history or examine the patient, direct them to obey the instructions – counsel the patient and explain the management.

PROMPT: "Doctor, does this mean that I have cancer?"

First, point out to Miss Bertram that this is NOT cancer.

½ mark

Explain low-grade changes:
- The changes are caused by infection with certain strains of the human papilloma-virus (HPV).
- HPV is very common in sexually active males and females.

- It causes two types of dysplastic (*pre*-cancerous) changes on the cervix – low-grade changes (CIN1) and high-grade changes (CIN2 and CIN3).
- Low-grade changes have a high chance of spontaneously resolving themselves (average time is 11 months, but can take up to 3 years). Two-thirds will resolve within a year.

3 marks

Appropriate management for low-grade abnormality is a repeat Pap smear in 12 months if patient is under 30 years old. If the patient is over 30 years old offer a repeat Pap smear in 6 months or an immediate colposcopy (Australian NHMRC Guidelines).

2 marks

- If the patient is a smoker it will increase the time to resolution, so they should be encouraged to quit.

½ mark

Q2
The essential point is that there is NO role for the HPV vaccine in this woman's current dysplasia as it is a prophylactic, not a therapeutic vaccine. However, she is still a candidate for the vaccine as it will protect her against future infection.

2 marks

Q3
Gardasil
- Protects against HPV strains 6 and 11 (cause genital warts), 16 and 18 (high-risk HPV types that together account for up to 70% of cervix cancer)

Cervarix
- Protects against HPV strains 16 and 18
- (*Extra mark*) For an extra mark the student will know that there is now evidence of cross-protection with some of the other high-risk strains.

2 marks (plus 1 bonus mark)

Q4
- Referral to a gynaecologist for a colposcopy

1 mark

Q5
Examination of the transformation zone of the cervix under magnification (the vagina and vulva should also be examined). The transformation zone is the area in which the dysplastic changes occur. Five per cent acetic acid is used to identify dysplastic changes (dysplastic cells stain white with acetic acid due to the different glycogen content). Abnormal areas are biopsied to confirm dysplasia. Lugols iodine can also be used to identify dysplastic areas and should be used to examine the vagina for evidence of dysplasia.

5 marks

Q6
- LLETZ or laser ablation

N.B. A cone biopsy is not indicated as there is no evidence of invasion on histology, and the changes do not extend up into the endocervical canal.

4 marks
20 marks total

Discussion
The student is expected to show a basic understanding of the diagnosis and management of cervical dysplasia, as well as knowledge of recent advances in prophylactic vaccines for HPV infection and cervical dysplasia.

The ability of the student to counsel a patient effectively regarding an abnormal Pap smear is tested in the first encounter.

A8   The student is expected to take an adequate history and discuss management of endometriosis.

Q1
History
- Regular periods every 28–30 days with 5 days bleeding. Not heavy. Last menstrual period 2 weeks ago. No inter-menstrual bleeding or bleeding after sexual intercourse
- Pain begins 2 days before onset of period and lasts 2 days into period. Started 2 years ago. No pain at other times, but occasional pain with intercourse. Pain can sometimes be so severe that she has to go home from her job as a secretary
- Pain relieved by Ponstan; occasionally needs Panadeine forte
- Sexually active – using condoms for contraception, one sexual partner
- No urinary or bowel symptoms. No abnormal vaginal discharge
- No past medical or surgical history
- Last Pap smear 12 months ago and normal

10 marks

Q2
- Chronic condition, classified as minimal, mild, moderate or severe
- Often occurrence of pain bears little correlation to severity of disease
- Management can be surgical and/or medical
- Surgery involves removal of deposits and normalising the anatomy
- Medical involves keeping endometriosis under control hormonally. Long-term use of COCP or Depo-Provera, short-term use of GnRH analogues
- If wants to be pregnant and infertile no evidence that hormonal treatment helps. Surgery of benefit particularly to normalise the anatomy. May need IVF if anatomy distorted or other factors present

10 marks
20 marks total

Discussion

Endometriosis is the presence of ectopic endometrial glands and stroma, and is one of the most common gynaecological problems. It is estimated that 7–10% of women have this condition and that it is present in 25–35% of infertile women. It usually presents in women between the ages of 30 and 45 years. Whether it presents as infertility, a pelvic mass, dysmenorrhoea, dyspareunia or non-cyclical pelvic pain, it can be an extremely debilitating disease.

The **diagnosis** should be suspected in a woman who presents with infertility, especially if she also complains of dysmenorrhoea that is getting worse with age and dyspareunia. It must be remembered that there is no correlation between the degree of pain and the severity of the endometriosis. There is no increase in the incidence of menstrual or ovulatory dysfunction, although there is some evidence that premenstrual spotting may occur in 50% of women with endometriosis.

On examination, the uterus may be retroverted and fixed and there may be tender nodules in the Pouch of Douglas (POD) and on the uterosacral ligaments.

The diagnosis of endometriosis must be made by **direct visualisation** of the lesions and/or their biopsy. Typical lesions are of blue/black powder-burn type, but they may also be red, vesicular, polypoid and non-pigmented. Adhesions and peritoneal windows may also be seen. The most common sites affected by endometriosis are the peritoneum of the uterosacrals, of the ovarian fossae and the POD, the ovaries, the bladder serosa, the sigmoid colon and the rectovaginal septum. Rarer locations are the vaginal mucosa, bladder wall, other abdominal and visceral peritoneum, abdominal scars, pleural cavity and lung parenchyma. Superficial endometriosis is more likely to be associated with infertility and deep endometriosis to be associated with pain.

The American Society for Reproductive Medicine (ASRM) scoring system is useful as an objective measure of disease severity and also for scoring treatment success, although its use is no longer widespread.

The rationale behind the usage of **hormones or medical therapy** in the management of endometriosis is that steroid hormones, particularly E, are major regulators of growth and function of endometriotic tissue. A lack of E, testosterone (T) or high dose P will produce atrophy.

One of the major treatment options is the COCP administered continuously. Pain will usually resolve within 3–6 months when total amenorrhoea occurs. **Progestogens** in high doses cause atrophy of endometriotic deposits. Depo-Provera is a good treatment choice. **Danazol** has been one of the most widely used therapies for endometriosis and is generally used for 6 months due to its hyper-androgenic side effects. It has been shown to cause an approximate 50% decrease in the endometriosis score after 6 months of treatment. This is mainly due to a decrease in the size and number of the implants. **Surgical castration** is the most effective treatment for endometriosis. On this is based the medical management of endometriosis using **GnRH analogues** (GnRHa), as these drugs will cause a reversible medical castration. All studies have universally shown an improvement in the endometriosis score by approximately 50% in approximately 80% of patients. The side effects of treatment are due to the hypo-oestrogenic state and are the same as those experienced by menopausal women: hot flushes, vaginal dryness, loss of libido and mood swings. The drugs are administered for 6 months due to the side effects as well as the negative impact on bone.

Surgery should attempt to normalise the anatomy and destroy or remove as much disease as possible. Care must be taken to prevent adhesions due to extensive surgery. Surgery may benefit minimal and mild disease if the patient is infertile, though this remains controversial. Normalising the anatomy will aid pregnancy. If fertility is no longer an issue radical surgery is the option. This involves hysterectomy and bilateral salpingo-oophorectomy.

The pain associated with endometriosis is effectively treated using medical and/or surgical management.

The **recurrence rate** of endometriosis is 5–20% per year with a reported cumulative rate of 40% after 5 years.

STUDENT OSCE B

B1 The student is expected to take an adequate history of the presenting problem and advise regarding emergency contraception, as well as the merits of using effective contraception.

Q1
History
- 27 years old
- Sexually active with 1 partner. Same partner for the last 4 years
- Usually use condoms but not always compliant. No other contraception used in past. The sex was consensual/unforced
- Periods generally occur every 30 days, lasting 5 days with no problems. LMP 2 weeks ago. Never used any hormones
- No past history – medical or surgical
- No family history
- No allergies, no medications, non-smoker, occasional alcohol
- Pap smear normal 12 months ago

8 marks total depending on completeness of history

Q2
'Postinor'– Laevonorgestrel (LNG) method. Must be used within 72 hours. 0.75 mg × 2 immediately or can be used as 1 tablet 12 hours apart. The former has better compliance. No prescription required. 1–2% failure. No

side effects as can occur with the 'Yuzpe method'. Must do pregnancy test if period delayed by 1 week.

3 marks total

The 'Yuzpe method' – 100 μg EE and 0.5 mg LNG administered 12 hours apart with an antiemetic due to vomiting that can occur with high dose of E. Must be within 72 hours. Failure rate 2–3%. Need to see a doctor for treatment. Must do pregnancy test if period delayed by 1 week.

3 marks total

Insertion of a copper IUD up to 5 days after unprotected intercourse. Failure rate is 2–3%. Should not be used in those at risk for PID or STIs. Can be used for ongoing contraception. Must do pregnancy test if period delayed by 1 week.

3 marks total

- Should discuss termination of pregnancy if a method fails.

1 mark

Q3
- Need to have adequate ongoing contraception so that not using emergency contraception as a method of contraception.

2 marks

20 marks total

Discussion

Emergency contraception is used if unprotected intercourse occurs or it is thought that another method has failed.

Currently the method of choice is '**Postinor**'. It can be obtained over the counter at the chemist. It needs to be used within 72 h of the event of unprotected intercourse. It is presented as 2 × 0.75 mg tablets. Compliance is better if both are taken immediately rather than 12 h apart. The failure rate is 1–2%.

The '**Yuzpe method**' is 100 μg ethinyl oestradiol (EE) and 0.5 mg LNG administered 12 h apart with an antiemetic. The failure rate is 2–3% if treatment is administered within 72 h. Its possible methods of action include inhibition of ovulation, effect on the luteal phase, effect on tubal transit time, embryotoxicity, induction of abortion and prevention of implantation by endometrial changes, the last being the most likely reason for success. Theoretically, the medication may be used up to the fourth or fifth day after unprotected intercourse.

The Task Force on Postovulatory Methods of Fertility Regulation, in a randomised controlled trial, compared LNG (0.75 mg 12 h apart) (Postinor-2) with the Yuzpe method started within 72 h of unprotected intercourse. They reported that the former method was more successful (1.1% vs 3.2%) and better tolerated.

An alternative method is the insertion of a copper IUD up to 5 days after unprotected intercourse. The failure rate is similarly 2–3%. This method prevents implantation. It should not be used in those at risk for PID or STIs. Its advantage is that it can be used for ongoing contraception.

Mifepristone (RU 486) (10 mg) is a most effective postcoital contraceptive agent. It is significantly more effective than the Yuzpe method (0% vs 2.62%) with fewer side effects. It can also be used up to 5 days after unprotected intercourse. When compared with the Yuzpe method it causes cycle prolongation. A Cochrane Review on emergency contraception reported that LNG 0.75 mg and RU486 offered the highest efficacy with acceptable side effects. However, RU486 caused a delay in the onset of menstruation, which caused anxiety in the women using this method. The WHO Research Group in Fertility Regulation published a randomised double-blind trial comparing the LNG method (1.5 mg as a single dose and 0.75 mg 12 h apart) with the use of RU486 at a single dose of 10 mg given within 5 days of intercourse. They showed no difference in pregnancy rates between groups, all being equally effective, and a low incidence of side effects. In the RU486 group there was a delay in the onset of menses. Given that there is no difference in efficacy between Postinor in divided doses versus 1 dose, the single dose regimen is preferable. A pregnancy test should be performed if the expected period does not occur within 3–4 weeks after taking emergency contraception. There is no evidence that failure of the LNG method is associated with an increase in congenital malformations or adverse pregnancy outcomes.

The woman should be offered an abortion if the method fails.

It is important that all women, especially teenagers, are well informed on the availability of emergency contraception. In Australia, Postinor is available over the counter, making it much more accessible, and ultimately this accessibility may decrease the number of unwanted pregnancies. Ready availability of emergency contraception does not lead to an increase in its use, an increase in unprotected sex or a decrease in the use of more reliable contraceptive methods (Marston et al 2005).

If appropriate, a patient requiring emergency contraception should be counselled regarding safe sex, and offered screening for sexually transmitted diseases. This is not appropriate in this case, as she is in a long-term monogamous relationship. It must always be considered a possibility that the unprotected sex was non-consensual (i.e. a rape), and this must be specifically asked for, as it may not be volunteered by the patient. Again, this is not the case with this patient. Finally, Pap smears must be discussed (should occur within one year of the first act of sexual intercourse, once over the age of 18 years), although our patient in this scenario has up-to-date, normal Pap smears.

References
Cheng L, Gulmezoglu A M, Van Oel C J et al 2004 Interventions for emergency contraception (Cochrane Review). The Cochrane Library, Issue 3. John Wiley, Chichester

Grou F, Rodrigues I 1994 The morning-after pill – How long after? American Journal of Obstetrics and Gynecology 171:1529

Marston C, Meltzer H, Majeed A 2005 Impact on contraceptive practice of making emergency hormonal contraception available over the counter in Great Britain: repeated cross sectional surveys. British Medical Journal 331:271

Speroff L, Darney P 1992 A clinical guide for contraception. Williams & Wilkins, Baltimore

Task Force on Postovulatory Methods of Fertility Regulation 1998 Randomised controlled trial of levonorgestrel versus the Yuzpe regimen of combined oral contraceptives for emergency contraception. Lancet 352:428

Who Research Group In Fertility Regulation 2002 Low dose Mifepristone and 2 regimens of levonorgestrel for emergency contraception. Lancet 360:1803

Yuzpe A A, Thurlow H J, Ramzy I et al 1974 Post coital contraception: a pilot study. Journal of Reproductive Medicine 13:53

B2 Q1

The student is expected to take a history and examine the patient, and then decide on a course of management.

History

- 25-year-old term (39 weeks gestation) primigravida
- Singleton pregnancy
- Antenatal testing all OK, apart from blood group B negative and group-B streptococcus +ve on high vaginal swab at 36 weeks
- No medical/surgical history
- No allergies
- Has been having 3 strong contractions in 10 minutes for last 2 hours
- Progress of labour in first stage adequate on vaginal assessments
- Liquor is clear, membranes ruptured 3 hours ago
- Has had one dose of pethidine 4 hours ago, and used nitrous gas up until started pushing
- Intermittent doppler of fetal heart shows fetal heart rate 130 bpm

6 marks, depending on completeness of history

Examination

- Clearly tired and distressed patient, lying supine
- PR 100, BP 130/85, temp 37.5 °C
- Abdominal Ex: term fundal height, contractions strong, longitudinal lie, no fetal head palpable above the pelvic brim, fetal heart rate 130 bpm
- Vaginal Ex: fully dilated cervix, cephalic, station +2 cm from ischial spines, position direct occiput-anterior, + caput, + moulding, liquor not seen, pelvis appears adequate

4 marks total

Management

- Diagnosis is prolonged second stage of labour

1 mark

- Patient needs forceps or ventouse delivery

1 mark

- CTG monitor to be applied
- Call paediatrician to be present at delivery

Q2
- Fully dilated cervix
- Cephalic presentation (can use in breech for aftercoming head, or in face mento-anterior)
- Station below ischial spines (high forceps, with station above spines, should never be attempted)
- No part of the fetal head palpable above the symphysis pubis
- Must be sure of correct position of the head
- No obvious cephalo-pelvic disproportion
- Empty bladder
- Adequate analgesia (in this situation, either pudendal nerve block, or epidural/spinal)
- Requires an episiotomy

½ mark for each (maximum 4 marks)

Q3
Maternal complications
- Short term
  - vaginal lacerations
  - perineal injuries/anal sphincter tears
  - extension of episiotomy
  - urinary retention
  - PPH
- Long term
  - incontinence of flatus/faeces (if damage to anal sphincter)
  - dyspareunia (if perineum scarred/injured)

½ mark for each (maximum of 2 marks)

Fetal complications
- Scalp/face lacerations/bruising
- Cephalhaematoma
- Subconjunctival haemorrhage
- Facial nerve injuries
- Skull fracture

½ mark for each (maximum of 2 marks)

Discussion
An OSCE station on forceps is a good way of determining if medical students have been spending time on the labour ward. It is usually poorly answered, despite its importance in obstetrics.

Instrumental vaginal delivery occurs in roughly 10–15% of all births in Victoria, with an even split between forceps and ventouse (vacuum) deliveries. Over the last 20 years the number of instrumental deliveries overall has declined, and the proportion of vacuum deliveries compared with forceps has increased. Presumably at least part of the decline in instrumental vaginal delivery can be accounted for by the steady and continuing rise in caesarean section rates in Victoria (from 15% in 1985 to 29.5% in 2004).

Types of forceps deliveries can be categorised according to the station of the presenting part (the fetal skull):

- Outlet forceps – fetal head is at or on the perineum, and visible without parting the labia.
- Low forceps – station +2 cm or more (below ischial spines).
- Mid-cavity forceps – station 0 cm (head 'engaged') to +2 cm).
- High forceps – no longer performed; fetal head above ischial spines.

The operator must be aware of a large caput (swelling of the fetal scalp) giving a falsely lower station than the fetal skull.

There are three types of forceps in use in Australia: the Neville-Barnes forceps (only to be used when in OA position; traction forceps only), the Kjelland forceps (rotational forceps), and the Wrigleys forceps (for outlet forceps and delivery of head at caesarean section only, as allows less traction than Neville-Barnes). At our university we have had OSCEs where the medical students were expected to identify the type of forceps as part of the station (see Figure 4.1 opposite), and point out both the parts of the forceps (blade, shank, lock, and handle), as well as the pelvic and cephalic curves.

Instrumental vaginal delivery is performed to shorten the second stage of labour and has a number of indications:

- Maternal: medical conditions benefiting from a short second stage (e.g. some cardiac disease), maternal exhaustion, prolonged second stage (greater than 2 hours in a nulliparous, and 1 hour in a parous woman; some operators allow an extra hour if an epidural is in use).
- Fetal: fetal distress (abnormal CTG, vaginal bleeding suspicious of an abruption), cord prolapse.

In the Neville-Barnes forceps delivery depicted in this station, the necessary pre-conditions are listed in the answer to question 2. The left blade of the forceps (to the maternal left pelvic side) should be inserted first, followed by the right blade. No more than three pulls should occur, each with an adequate uterine contraction, and coordinated with maternal pushing. If there is the suspicion that the forceps may be difficult, a trial of forceps in theatre, so that conversion to a caesarean section can be performed rapidly, is appropriate.

In listing the possible complications of the forceps delivery, the better answers will be divided into maternal and fetal categories, as well as short- and long-term complications.

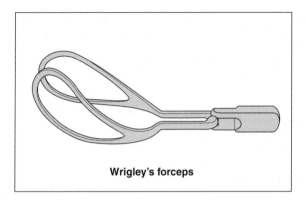

Wrigley's forceps

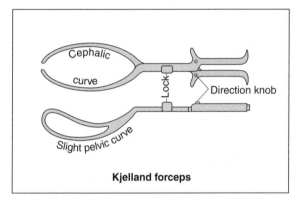

Kjelland forceps

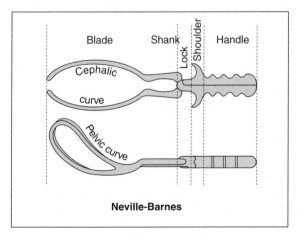

Neville-Barnes

Figure 4.1   Different types and features of forceps (obstetric forceps from Pairman *et al.* 2006 Midwifery: preparation for practice, Elsevier, Sydney. Based on J Oats & S Abraham 2004, Llewellyn-Jones Fundamentals of obstetrics and gynaecology, 8th edn, Elsevier, Edinburgh)

B3 The student is expected to take an adequate history of the presenting problem and ask relevant questions about key examination findings. They are also expected to ask for appropriate diagnostic tests and counsel the patient regarding treatment options for the presenting complaint (the dual problems of irregular cycles and hirsutism/excessive hair growth).

Q1
- 27 years old
- Menarche 12 years
- Periods have always been about 3–6 monthly. Lasting 5 days. No problems. LMP 2 weeks ago. Never used any hormones
- Never sexually active
- Acne as a teenager
- Hirsutism on chin (plucks hair), around nipples (no treatment), on abdomen (waxes) and waxes legs every 3–4 weeks. Problem since menarche
- If asks for symptoms of virilism such as voice deepening, change to body shape, clitoral enlargement, balding – not present
- Size 16–18; has always struggled with weight
- No past history – medical or surgical
- Mother has type II diabetes, father has hypertension
- No allergies, no medications, non-smoker, occasional alcohol

10 marks total, depending on completeness of history

Q2
- BMI 32
- BP 110/75
- Terminal hair on upper lip, chin, around nipples and thick hair over lower abdomen. If asks for Ferriman-Gallwey score 18
- Acanthosis nigricans on nape of neck
- No pink abdominal striae
- Other examination normal

5 marks total (1 mark for each point of examination asked for)

Q3
- FSH, LH, prolactin, testosterone, DHEAS, TSH
- Pelvic ultrasound
- Glucose tolerance test, lipid profile

3 marks total (½ mark for each of the above ordered)

Q4
Weight loss and exercise are extremely important, both for resolution of immediate symptoms and reduction of the risk of diabetes and cardiovascular disease later in life.

To control hirsutism and regulate cycle:

- Cosmetic measures, such as shaving, depilatory creams, electrolysis
  1 mark
- Hormonal treatments, such as OCP (Yasmin or Diane 35) ±
  antiandrogen such as Aldactone
  1 mark
  20 marks total

Discussion

Polycystic ovarian syndrome (PCOS) is the most common reproductive endocrine disorder in women of reproductive age, with a prevalence ranging from 5–10%. It is the most common cause of anovulatory infertility. It is a **heterogenous** condition with various combinations of symptoms and signs, such as:

- menstrual irregularities, including oligomennorrhoea or amenorrhoea
- infertility
- androgen excess
- obesity, although 10% of women with PCOS are of normal weight
- insulin resistance with compensatory hyperinsulinaemia.

The **diagnosis** of PCOS can be difficult. The Rotterdam Consensus on Diagnostic Criteria for PCOS (2003) states that a diagnosis of PCOS must include two out of three of the following:

- Oligo- and/or amenorrhoea (<8 uterine bleedings/year).
- Clinical and/or biochemical signs of hyperandrogenism.
- Polycystic ovaries on ultrasound.

Other aetiologies (e.g. congenital adrenal hyperplasia, androgen-secreting tumours, Cushing's syndrome) must be excluded.

The older NIH criteria (1990) stated that a diagnosis was made in a woman with:

- irregular periods
- clinical or biochemical hyperandrogenism
- exclusion of other causes.

Each of these criteria has problems. The Rotterdam criteria may overdiagnose the condition and the NIH criteria may underdiagnose the condition. The diagnosis is still a work in progress.

Polycystic ovaries on ultrasound can be diagnosed in up to 20% of all women, although with the recent change to the number of follicles counted in each ovary up to 50% may have PCO. The ultrasound diagnosis of PCO is defined as the presence of 12 or more follicles of 2–9 mm diameter in at least one ovary with or without increased ovarian stromal volume (>10 mL).

Clinical signs of hyperandrogenism

Clinical signs of hyperandrogenism include:

- acne
- hirsutism: excessive growth of hair, or growth of hair in atypical areas, e.g. face, breast, abdomen

- Ferriman-Gallwey Scoring System 11 areas with maximal score of 4 in each area
- male-pattern baldness
- virilisation: deepening of voice
- clitoral hypertrophy
- breast atrophy
- increased muscle bulk.

The **aetiology** of PCOS is unknown. It has a familial tendency, suggesting a genetic basis for its inheritance. A woman has a 50% chance of developing PCOS if she has an affected sister. While this could reflect autosomal dominant inheritance, it is more likely that there is an interaction of environmental factors with a small number of causative genes. There is some evidence that PCOS may manifest itself as early as in utero, with an increased risk of IUGR and post-term birth. In utero androgen exposure has also been associated with masculine finger length patterns, as well as childhood hyperinsulinaemia and premature pubarche. PCOS is often, but not always, triggered by weight gain, implicating insulin resistance and hyperinsulinaemia as causal factors. Similarly, by losing weight/reducing fat mass, overweight PCOS patients can increase their tissue insulin sensitivity and restore menstrual cyclicity. Hyperinsulinaemia and insulin resistance may act in genetically predisposed women to unmask latent abnormalities in steroid production. In vitro, insulin also stimulates androgen synthesis in theca cells and decreases SHBG, increasing free androgen availability.

The hyperandrogenic milieu of PCOS results in an increased pituitary sensitivity to GnRH stimulation. This results in higher LH secretory episodes in response to each GnRH secretory burst. LH luteinises theca cells, thus producing further testosterone and androstenedione. These androgens are aromatised to oestrogens, and also inhibit the production of SHBG, resulting in a reduction of bound oestrogen and testosterone.

Long-term health risks

There are several long-term health risks associated with PCOS:

Insulin resistance

- Up to 50% with PCOS
- Women with PCOS have a 3–7× risk of developing type II diabetes
- Occurs in up to 75% of obese and 30% of non-obese PCOS women
- Risk factors for type II diabetes in PCOS patients include:
  – obesity
  – family history of type II diabetes
  – anovulation
- Progression of impaired glucose tolerance (IGT) can be delayed by lifestyle and pharmacological intervention.

Cardiovascular disease

PCOS patients have increased risk factors for cardiac disease:

- Obesity
- IGT/type II diabetes

- Markers of abnormal vascular function – increased CRP, t-PAI
- Dyslipidaemia – increased triglycerides, reduced HDL
- Hypertension – 3× risk
  However, limited epidemiological studies have shown no direct evidence of an increased incidence of mortality from coronary heart disease, although the incidence of stroke is slightly increased.

Endometrial hyperplasia and cancer

PCOS patients are at increased risk of endometrial hyperplasia as a result of chronic anovulation and unopposed oestrogen exposure. Hyperandrogenaemia and elevated IGF (insulin-like growth factor-1) concentrations are also implicated as risk factors for the development of endometrial cancer in PCOS patients.

There is a theoretical increased risk (up to 4×) of endometrial carcinoma in PCOS patients. However, while PCOS is associated with risk factors for endometrial cancer, it does not necessarily follow that there is an increased incidence or mortality from endometrial cancer. Nevertheless, women with longstanding anovulation (<1/4–6 months) and a thickened endometrium on ultrasound should have an endometrial biopsy to exclude malignancy.

Pregnancy risks

Some studies suggest PCOS patients are at increased risk of gestational diabetes, recurrent miscarriage and IUGR. However, other studies suggest that the increased weight/BMI is the main risk factor, rather than PCOS per se.

Other

Increased risk of:
- sleep apnoea
- endometriosis
- breast cancer

Taking a history

When seeing a woman with PCOS these are the key points in taking a history:
- Menstrual pattern – from menarche to present
- Hyperandrogenism – acne, hirsutism, alopecia
  N.B. rapid onset/progression – suggestive of androgen secreting tumour
- Fertility/infertility
- Lifestyle – diet and exercise
- Recent weight gain
- Family history
- Medications – androgens, phenytoin, diazoxide as cause of hirsutism
- Smoker – CVS risk factor

Examination

The key examination points include:
- general – BP, BMI
- thyroid – goitre
- CVS

- visual fields – pituitary adenoma
- hirsutism and male pattern baldness – Ferriman-Gallwey scale normal < 8 for caucasian women
- acne
- virilisation – deep voice, clitoromegaly, android body shape, increased muscle mass, breast atrophy
- Cushing's syndrome – striae, central obesity, moon-like facies, buffalo hump, hypertension
- *Acanthosis nigricans* – associated with severe insulin resistance
- abdomen – masses, e.g. androgen-secreting tumours
- pelvic, Pap smear if required

Investigations

- PCOS patients with oligo/anovulation are typically normo-gonadotropic and normo-oestrogenic, although LH concentrations are frequently elevated (>95th centile in ~60% of PCOS patients) due to increased amplitude and frequency of LH pulses. An LH:FSH ratio >2 can aid in the diagnosis, but a normal ratio does not exclude the condition. By the same token, an LH <3 in a woman with amenorrhoea makes the diagnosis of hypogonadism.
- Total testosterone: may be elevated (>1.5 nmol/L)
- SHBG: may be reduced
- Free androgen index: ratio of testosterone: SHBG often increased in PCOS
- DHEAS: can have mild isolated increase in PCOS, often greatly elevated (>2x normal) with androgen-secreting tumours from the adrenal
- Prolactin: hyperprolactinaemia may be associated with oligo/anovulation. Hyperandrogenism may be associated with mildly elevated prolactin
- TFTs: thyroid disease may be associated with weight gain and menstrual irregularities, and is not uncommon in females of reproductive age
- 17-OHP: to exclude 21-hydroxylase deficient non-classical CAH. This may be evident clinically by rapid onset of hirsutism and virilism at puberty
- GTT: Measurements of fasting insulin and insulin tolerance tests are not recommended
- Fasting lipid profile

Management of PCOS

Non-pharmacological methods

Weight reduction and other lifestyle measures (e.g. diet and exercise)
   – This is the most important intervention in an overweight or obese woman with PCOS. Some studies have shown that a 5% loss of weight can restore ovulation in up to 90% of PCOS patients, with 60% becoming pregnant within 18 months.

– This can be facilitated by enrolling patients into a lifestyle program.
• Hair removal
  – Cosmetic measures such as bleaching, waxing, shaving, depilatory
    cream, electrolysis and laser

Medical methods

Combined oral contraceptive pill (COCP)

If a PCOS patient does not want pregnancy, administration of a COCP may
have the following benefits:
• Control of endometrial growth with prevention of endometrial
  hyperplasia and carcinoma.
• Inhibition of excess ovarian androgen production, with reduction in
  hirsutism, acne, and so on.
• Improvement in HDL:LDL with low-androgenic gestagens
  (N.B. Triglycerides typically increase with COCP use.)
• COCPs inhibit folliculogenesis, as a result of suppression of pituitary
  gonadotrophin production.
• COCPs also reduce free circulating androgens by:
  – stimulating the synthesis of sex-hormone binding globulin
    (oestrogen effect)
  – inhibiting adrenal steroidogenesis (DHEAS) (progesterone effect).

A daily dose of 30–35 ug of Ethinyl Estradiol (EE) guarantees sufficient
suppression of ovarian follicular activity, as well as effective stimulation
of SHBG production. The first choice of gestagen should be one with low
androgenic potential (e.g. gestodene, desogestrel, norgestrel). Cyproterone
acetate and drosperinone are specific antiandrogens and COCPs containing
these as the progestogen components should be the first choice if possible.
Yasmin, which contains drosperinone, may be a better choice than Diane 35
(which contains cyproterone acetate), as the latter can often cause
bloating.

*N.B. Caution should be taken using COCPs in patients who are very obese,
smokers, hypertensive or hypercholesterolaemic. If a woman is >35 years old
and smokes, the COCP is an absolute contraindication.*

Progestogens
• Main clinical benefit is to ensure a regular withdrawal bleed when
  taken cyclically (e.g. 12 days per month)
• Progestogens inhibit: gonadotropin stimulation of ovarian androgen
  production, 5α-reductase activity in the skin and adrenal androgen
  production.
• All of the above, however, only occur at higher doses than are given
  for inducing a withdrawal bleed (e.g. Provera 10 mg). The Mirena IUD
  also provides excellent endometrial protection and can be used as a
  treatment in the PCOS patient with endometrial hyperplasia.

Anti-androgens
There is some evidence showing a more pronounced and faster improvement of skin androgenic symptoms, especially hirsutism, using a combination of COCP with anti-androgens. Need a trial for at least 6 months to see an effect.

As their mechanism of action (blocking the androgen receptor) is different from COCP, they can act synergistically with COCPs. They are also prescribed with COCP for contraception, as anti-androgens have a teratogenic effect on male fetuses. The two most commonly used drugs are aldactone and cyproterone acetate.

Management of infertility

Ovulation induction (OI)
A Cochrane review concludes that either Metformin or clomiphene citrate can be used as first-line agents in ovulation induction, and combination therapy is more effective than single-agent therapy. However, this is a subject that continues to be researched and these recommendations may change.

* OI with gonadotrophins
* Requires daily injections of recombinant FSH, with incremental increases in dose until there is a follicular response.

References

Cattrall F, Vollenhoven B, Weston G 2005 Anatomical evidence for in utero androgen exposure in women with polycystic ovarian syndrome. Fertility and Sterility 84(6):1689–1692

Harborne L, Fleming R, Lyall H, Norman J, Sattar N 2003 Descriptive review of the evidence for the use of Metformin in polycystic ovarian syndrome. The Lancet 361(9372):1894–1901

Kjotrod S, von During V, Carlsen S 2004 Metformin treatment before IVF/ICSI in women with PCOS; a prospective, randomised, double-blinded study. Human Reproduction 19(6):1315–1322

Kovacs G 2005 Polycystic ovaries and polycystic ovarian syndrome. Obstetrics and Gynecology 7(4):41–43

Pillay O, Te Fong L, Crow J et al 2006 The association between polycystic ovaries and endometrial cancer. Human Reproduction 21(4):924–929

Speroff L, Glass R, Kase N 1999 Clinical gynaecologic endocrinology and infertility, 6th edn. Williams & Wilkins, Lippincott

B4 Q1

History
* 29-year-old G3P1 at 39/40 gestation
* Woke up 6 hours ago with a gush of fluid into the bed. Soaked the bedsheets.
* No contractions
* Fetal movements felt by patient
* Past obstetric history: normal vaginal delivery at term 3 years ago, uncomplicated pregnancy; 1 miscarriage at 8 weeks last year, uncomplicated, treated with a suction curette

- Current pregnancy uneventful – no hypertension or gestational diabetes
- Blood group A +ve; GBS negative (tested at 36/40)
- No medical problems
- Past Hx: suction curette last year, nil else
- No family Hx of note
- No medications, NKA
- Lives with husband and 3 year-old daughter, full-time mother, non-smoker, non-drinker

4 marks

Examination
- BP 130/80, PR 80, RR 16, T 37
- Abdominal Ex: non-tender uterus, longitudinal lie, cephalic presentation, head 3/5 above the pelvic brim, fetal movements felt, fetal heart +ve with Doppler
- Sterile speculum Ex: clear liquor draining from cervical os, no cord present, cervix multi-os and central, Amnicator +ve if tested for

4 marks
Subtract 1 mark if performs vaginal examination

Investigation/management
- CTG – reactive normal heart trace

PROMPTS by examiner: "Can I go home, doctor? If so, is there anything I have to watch out for?"

Management options
1 Induction of labour, either immediately or the next day – need to confirm forewaters with forceps, and start IV Syntocinon, with continuous CTG monitoring; once prolonged rupture of membranes (>18 hours) will need IV antibiotics (penicillin)
2 Conservative management – await onset of normal labour

For conservative management (can wait up to 96 hours for onset of labour), the following are needed:
- Twice-daily temperature measurement by patient
- Adequate fetal movements (>10 per day)
- Daily normal CTG until in labour
- No change to colour of liquor (no meconium)
- No fever or abdominal pain
- Oral antibiotics (augmentin or amoxicillin + potassium clavulanate)
- Will need IV antibiotics in labour (penicillin) due to prolonged ruptured membranes
- After 96 hours, recommend induction of labour even if the clinical situation is unchanged

2 marks for describing options
½ mark for each condition necessary for conservative Mx (2 marks maximum)

Q2

- Likely meconium in the liquor
- Needs to have a CTG – if suitable/normal, needs to have induction of labour
- IV Syntocinon after confirmation of ruptured forewaters
- Continuous CTG monitoring
- IV penicillin to mother (prolonged ruptured membranes)
- Suctioning of the airway/trachea of the fetus after delivery of the head

1 mark for each (4 marks maximum)

Q3

- Fever
- Tender abdomen/uterus
- Change in colour of liquor from clear (can check pads)
- Raised C-reactive protein
- Rise in white cell count
- CTG with fetal tachycardia (>160 bpm)

1 mark for each (4 marks maximum)

20 marks total

Discussion

Between 6% and 12% of pregnant women experience membrane rupture prior to the onset of labour. In only 2–3% of pregnant women will the rupture of membranes occur prior to 37 weeks gestation.

The management must be negotiated with the patient in this instance, but once cord presentation/prolapse, chorioamnionitis and fetal distress are excluded it is reasonable to institute conservative management, as the patient wishes, so long as the woman adheres to a strict monitoring for signs of infection or fetal compromise.

In the third question, the student is expected to list the signs, symptoms and investigation findings in a preterm pregnancy with chorioamnionitis.

B5 Q1

History

- Mrs Broadbent, a 49-year-old woman
- "My clothes have been getting tighter over the past 2–3 months."
- "I can feel a lump in the lower abdomen."
- No nausea or vomiting
- Sensation of early satiety
- Recent reflux
- Urinary frequency and the sensation that the bladder is always full
- Recent episodes of diarrhoea
- Para 3 (3 NVDs, children 12, 14 and 18 years old)
- Periods stopped 2 years ago; no hormone therapy
- Last Pap smear 12/12 ago (always normal)
- Laparoscopic tubal ligation at 42 years old

- NKA Nil medications
- Family Hx: adopted, doesn't know family history
- Lives with husband and 3 children; works in family hardware store; smokes 15 cigarettes per day, occasional alcohol

5 marks, depending on completeness of history

Q2
Examination
- BMI 24
- Head and neck normal; no lymph nodes palpable
- Cardiorespiratory Ex: dual heart sounds, nil added; dull to percussion in R lung base
- Breast Ex: normal
- Abdominal Ex: distended, with clinical ascites; firm mass above symphysis; no groin nodes
- Vulva/vagina: normal
- Speculum: normal parous cervix
- PV/PR Ex: firm irregular mass, separate to uterus; some mobility

4 marks, depending on completeness

Q3
Investigations
- FBE, urea + electrolytes + creatinine, liver function tests
- Tumour markers: CA125, CA15.3, CA19.9, LDH, CEA
- CXR
- Pelvic ultrasound scan
- CT scan chest, abdomen, pelvis

3 marks (½ mark for each up to 3 marks)

Q4
Examiner plays the role of the patient
Need to explain to the patient clearly and simply that the scan shows tumours on both ovaries, with high probability of cancer, as they are complex masses, tumour marker CA125 is markedly elevated, and there is ascites.

Acknowledge that this is a shock.

The first step in treatment is referral to a gynaecological oncologist for surgery.

PROMPT: "Has the cancer spread, Doctor?" "Will I die from this?"

Need to be honest and straightforward with the patient.

"The CT scan does suggest that the cancer has spread beyond the ovaries, but this is the case for the majority of women in your situation. The important thing is that we get on with your treatment promptly."

Will need surgery for cytoreduction of tumour load, followed by chemotherapy.

4 marks for correct information
3 marks for appropriate sensitivity in counselling patient
20 marks total

Discussion
In this OSCE, not only is the student expected to arrive at the likely diagnosis by information gained from the history, examination and investigations, but they are also expected to deal sensitively with how they impart the bad news to the patient. Marks are assigned to the appropriate manner in dealing with the patient's reaction to the likely diagnosis.

B6 Q1
- Identify that the BP is higher than acceptable
- Identify that 2+ protein is not normal
- Diagnosis may be consistent with pre-eclampsia

1 mark each (2 marks maximum)

Proceed to take a history

History
Medical history
- Booking blood pressure (120/70)
- Any prior diagnosis of essential or secondary hypertension (nil)
- Any anti-hypertensives prescribed whether prior to or during pregnancy (nil)
- Family history of pre-eclampsia (yes: sister and mother)
- Any medical illnesses known to predispose to pre-eclampsia: connective tissue disease, IDDM (no)

1 mark each (3 marks maximum)

Current symptoms
- Headache
- Visual disturbance
- Epigastric pain
- Edema
- Fetal wellbeing: Presence or absence of fetal movements

½ mark each (2 marks maximum)

Examination
- Repeat BP (160/100)
- Assessment of symphysio-fundal height (38 cm)
- Fetal lie/presentation: longitudinal lie, cephalic presentation
- Presence of fetal heart (present, 140 bpm)
- Vaginal assessment of cervix: Bishop score (unfavourable – would need Prostin for induction of labour)

½ mark each (2 marks maximum)

Q2
- Identify need for admission
- Identify need for investigations to assess severity of PET
- Identify need to assess the fetus for compromise due to PET
- Identify need for delivery if PET confirmed
- Identify possible need for anti-hypertensives

1 mark each (4 marks maximum)

Possible investigations

Maternal
- FBE
- U/E/Cr
- LFTs
- Coag screen
- Uric acid
- 24-hour urine collection OR spot protein/creatinine ratio

1 mark each (3 marks maximum)

Fetal
- CTG
- Ultrasound for growth
- Assessment of liquour volume
- Doppler of the umbilical artery

½ mark each (2 marks maximum)

Possible treatment
- Anti-hypertensives: Aldomet/Labetalol/Nifedipine

1 mark

Possible further management
- Induction of labour

1 mark
20 marks total

Discussion
Pre-eclampsia is a common condition of pregnancy affecting 5–10% of primigravidas. It is defined as:
- blood pressure >140/90 mmHg, in a woman with normal BP prior to pregnancy
- proteinuria > 0.3 g per 24 hours
- peripheral oedema.

Given the common nature of the condition, as well as the potentially disastrous consequences for mother and fetus if the diagnosis is missed or delayed, students are expected to have a thorough knowledge of the condition and its investigation and treatment. Refer to standard obstetrics textbooks for more information.

B7

The student is expected to take an adequate history and advise regarding the use of hormone therapy, its benefits and risks.

Q1
History
- 54 years old
- 3 pregnancies and 3 children born by vaginal delivery; healthy
- No periods for 12 months; prior to that about every 1–3 months for 2 years and prior to that regular
- Hot flushes and night sweats for the past 18 months; getting worse; difficulty sleeping, tired, irritable; vaginal dryness and pain with intercourse
- Only had 1 partner; used condoms in the past
- No past history – medical or surgical
- Family history: mother developed breast cancer at age of 54 years
- No allergies, no medications, non-smoker, occasional alcohol
- Pap smear 6 months ago; normal mammogram 9 months ago
- Works as a secretary

8 marks

Q2
- HT given as a combined preparation with both E and P
- Can be given continuously as she has had no period for 12 months
- Advantage of continuous use is that no return of bleeding, but may get irregular bleeding/spotting
- Early side effects include breast tenderness, nausea and headaches

4 marks

Q3
Benefits
- Effective relief of symptoms, including vaginal symptoms
- Bone protection and treatment for osteopaenia and osteoporosis
- May protect against bowel cancer

Risks
- Deep venous thrombosis
- After 5 years slight increase in breast cancer, heart attack and stroke

8 marks
20 marks total

Discussion
Menopause is defined as the cessation of menses for at least 1 year and usually occurs between the ages of 48 and 55 years. Over the centuries there has been no change in the time of menopause. As the population ages and lifespans increase, most women in developed countries can expect to spend at least one-third of their lives in menopause.

The most common symptoms are hot flushes and night sweats; these occur in over 85% of menopausal women. They are more likely to occur at night and may precede the menopause by a number of years. They may last 5 years after the final cessation of periods, although in 10% of women these symptoms persist. Other symptoms include vaginal dryness, skin changes such as drying and thinning, a variety of psychological symptoms including loss of memory, anxiety, mood swings and irritability, a decrease in libido and a lack of energy. Other common complaints include headaches, dizziness, palpitations, insomnia and myalgias. Depression is not caused by menopause, but transitory depression may occur when a woman experiences a prolonged menopausal transition (at least 27 months). This is thought to be due to the presence of symptoms.

While some women experience no symptoms at all, 50–60% of women seek help in dealing with the problems of menopause.

Risks of HT

Most women use hormone therapy (HT) to relieve symptoms. Oestrogen can also be used for both the prevention and treatment of osteoporosis and its use is based on data from randomised controlled trials. Oestrogen therapy reduces the risk of osteoporosis and increases bone density by approximately 5–10%. The risk of hip and arm fractures is reduced by 50–60% and the risk of vertebral deformation by 90%, based on epidemiological data. It has also been shown to be protective against colorectal cancer. This is based on both observational studies, as well as the WHI trial.

One of the risks of HT is breast cancer. Overall, the administration of HT is associated with a very small risk of breast cancer after 5 years of use based on epidemiological data as well as the WHI trial. In this trial the excess number of breast cancers that developed was 8 in the treated group (10,000 women) with no increase in mortality. There was no increase in breast cancer in the women on ET alone. The risk of endometrial hyperplasia and cancer is associated with the administration of E without P in women with a uterus. The risk increases substantially with prolonged duration of use (more than tenfold after more than 10 years) and the risk persists for several years after discontinuation (over 5 years).

Women using HT are also at risk of thromboembolic disease. This is in the order of two to three times the background risk. The WHI trial has also shown that HT should not be used for primary prevention of heart attack, and previous studies have shown that HT cannot be used for secondary prevention of heart attack. The WHI trial demonstrated that after 5 years of use of HT there were 8 extra cases of heart attack in 10,000 women compared with women using a placebo.

The regimen of HT depends on the presence or absence of a uterus. If the uterus is absent only E need be given. However, if the uterus is present then P therapy needs to be administered for at least 10 days of each month. The disadvantage of this mode of treatment is that a withdrawal bleed will occur on cessation of the P treatment. To prevent this both E and P can be administered daily.

B8 Q1

History

- Mrs Tran is a 33-year-old Vietnamese woman
- Unplanned singleton pregnancy, but wants to keep the baby
- 10 weeks gestation by an ultrasound 1 week ago, as well as by dates
- G2P1 – had a normal vaginal delivery of a boy 3 years ago (he is well)
- Not on folate/multivitamins, and not aware of rubella status
- Mild nausea, no other pregnancy symptoms
- No screening tests yet
- No relevant gynaecological history. Never had a Pap smear
- No past medical/surgical Hx
- No relevant family Hx
- Non-smoker, non-drinker, married and lives with husband and son; both she and her husband are currently looking for work
- No allergies or medications
- Jaundice started 3 days ago, noticed by GP when she went for a pregnancy test for her delayed period; no previous episodes of jaundice
- Associated mild, right upper quadrant discomfort
- Urine has been darker of late, and some pale diarrhoea
- No known history of gallstones or hepatitis. No past IVDU

6 marks

Examination

- Vitals: PR 80, BP 110/70, T 37°C
- Mild jaundice (skin/sclera)
- FWT: no protein/glucose
- Cardiorespiratory Ex: normal
- Abdominal Ex: slight RUQ tenderness, no masses
- VE – 10/40 uterus, anteverted, no adnexal masses
- Speculum: normal cervix (can take Pap smear at this stage)

2 marks

PROMPT: "Do you need to organise any tests, doctor?"

Investigations

1 Routine antenatal investigations
   Blood group and antibodies, FBE, rubella serology, TPHA, MSU(M/C/S), HIV serology
   Consider/offer Down syndrome screening
2 LFTs
3 Hep A, B, C serology
4 Upper abdominal ultrasound looking for gallstones

5 marks

Q2

- Mrs Tran has evidence of acute Hepatitis B infection
- Should involve a gastroenterologist/infectious disease physician in management

- Notifiable disease to Health Department
- Should test for Hep B and vaccinate husband and son against Hepatitis B if they are negative. Warn against sexual intercourse and sharing of toothbrushes until husband is vaccinated

2 marks

Management of pregnancy
- No risk of fetal abnormality from infection
- Need to consider health of both mother and baby

Mother
- Check LFTs regularly throughout pregnancy (at least weekly until clinically improved, and then monthly)
- Closer to delivery, if LFTs still abnormal, check INR (risk of bleeding if clotting factors from liver reduced)

2 marks

PROMPT: "How do I stop my baby getting Hepatitis B, doctor? Would a caesarean section help?"

Baby
- Staff to exercise universal precautions at delivery. Avoid fetal scalp blood sampling and instrumental delivery if possible
- Needs to have Hep B passive and active immunisation with Hep B immunoglobulins and Hep B vaccine respectively, after birth to prevent transmission of Hep B virus
- Further vaccinations at 2, 4 and 12 months after birth
- Need serological testing at 12 months with paediatrician

There is no evidence that caesarean section lowers the risk of HBV transmission compared with vaginal delivery.

3 marks
20 marks total

Discussion

In this OSCE the student must deal with a jaundiced patient in the first trimester of pregnancy. The main differential diagnosis in such a patient includes:
- alcohol and drug-induced hepatitis (ruled out on history in this patient)
- gallstones/obstructive jaundice (ruled out with abdominal ultrasound)
- viral hepatitis – Hepatitis A, B or C (assessed by serology).

There are other rarer causes, but there is nothing in the patient's history to suggest these.

This is a very different scenario to jaundice presenting in late pregnancy, when cholestasis of pregnancy, acute fatty liver of pregnancy, and HELLP syndrome complicating pre-eclampsia would be important differential diagnoses. This case is of early pregnancy, and these diagnoses are not relevant here.

It is important to remember to perform the routine antenatal testing, as well as testing for a cause of jaundice.

In this case of acute (or acute on chronic) Hepatitis B infection, the management should include general measures, as well as consideration of maternal health and prevention of vertical transmission to the baby. Marks are allocated for stating relevant important negatives, such as the fact that there is no risk of fetal abnormalities and that a caesarean section will not prevent vertical transmission.

STUDENT OSCE C

C1 Q1

The student is not expected to take a history or examine the patient. They should be directed to counsel the patient directly about risks if they start to take a history.

Antenatal – maternal
- Miscarriage rate increased
- Hyperemesis gravidarum (both increased rate and severity)
- Iron-deficiency anaemia
- Exaggerated general symptoms of pregnancy (e.g. backache and gastro-oesophageal reflux)
- Antepartum haemorrhage
- Gestational hypertension
- Pre-eclampsia
- Gestational diabetes
- Premature rupture of membranes
- Premature delivery (both iatrogenic due to fetal or maternal condition, as well as due to increased uterine distension)

Antenatal – fetal
- Congenital anomalies
- Intrauterine growth retardation (IUGR)
- Perinatal mortality rate
- Growth discordance (not associated with twin–twin transfusion syndrome)

Intrapartum
- Increased need for operative delivery (forceps, breech extraction of second twin, caesarean section), with increased risk of trauma to mother and baby

Postpartum
- Post-partum haemorrhage (due to uterine distension)
- Breastfeeding difficulties (need supply for two babies)
- Financial difficulties
- Postnatal depression (partly due to increased stressors and increased intervention needed at birth)

Problems unique to monochorionic twins
- Twin–twin transfusion syndrome (TTTS) (15–20% of monochorionic twins)

12 marks (depending on completeness)

Q2
- TTTS can only occur with monochorionic twins
- Clinical signs of TTTS: rapid abdominal/uterine distension, reduced ability to palpate fetal parts (massive polyhydramnios)
- Ultrasound screening every 2–4 weeks from 24–28 weeks gestation is indicated to look for signs of TTTS. Signs of TTTS on ultrasound include:
  – growth discordance between the twins
  – polyhydramnios (recipient twin), and oligohydramnios/anhydramnios (donor twin)

4 marks (depending on completeness)

Q3
- Twins should have no fetal compromise/distress
- Should be near term
- First (lead) twin must be cephalic (presentation of second twin is not important, as can perform internal cephalic version and breech extraction of second twin)
- Delivery should be in a hospital, with an experienced obstetrician, paediatrician and anaesthetist available
- Epidural/spinal
- Intravenous access
- Continuous monitoring of both twins with cardiotocograph

4 marks (depending on completeness)
20 marks total

Discussion
The key to the first, and largest, part of this OSCE is to have an organised approach to dividing up the risks, so that you are less likely to forget problems that are increased or unique to twins. A suggestion is to divide the problems into antenatal (both maternal and fetal problems to be considered separately), intrapartum and postpartum problems, with an additional category of problems unique to this twin pregnancy (i.e. TTTS).

About 3.5% of all births in the state of Victoria are twins, with about one-third of them resulting from reproductive treatment (ovulation induction and IVF). Twins are risky pregnancies. Twin babies have roughly a four-fold risk of perinatal mortality (much of this due to the increased risk of prematurity: only 6% of singleton pregnancies are less than 37 weeks gestation at birth, compared with over 50% of twins). Twin pregnancies are more than twice as likely to be delivered by caesarean section than a singleton pregnancy. The many increased risks are listed in the answer to question 1. The best students will demonstrate lateral thinking and also consider the social and psychological problems increased in parents of twin pregnancies (see answer to question 2).

It is extremely important to determine chorionicity (number of placentas) of a twin pregnancy, which can only be accurately determined by a first trimester ultrasound examination of the placental mass(es). After the first trimester the placental masses – even of a dichorionic pregnancy – fuse, making the differentiation of a monochorionic from a dichorionic pregnancy difficult. The shared vasculature of twins with a single placenta can result in imbalances of flow, with the twin that receives a greater proportion of blood flow gradually growing relatively larger, and with a greater amount of surrounding amniotic liquor. TTTS (which occurs in about 15% of monochorionic twin pregnancies) should be managed in a specialist unit, usually of a tertiary hospital, where close monitoring, treatment and delivery options can be decided.

While some obstetricians will perform a caesarean section on all twin pregnancies, the prevailing view in Australia in 2007 is still that vaginal birth of twins is acceptable if the criteria listed in the answer to question 3 are met. At present, it is unacceptable to deliver twins vaginally if the presentation of the first twin is not cephalic, or head first. This view may change with the result of an ongoing large randomised trial of vaginal birth versus caesarean section for twins.

C2 Q1

History

- 24-year-old woman in first pregnancy
- Planned, spontaneous pregnancy. Roughly 9 weeks since last menstrual period
- Was not on folate, and rubella status unknown. No antenatal investigations to date (has an appointment at a public antenatal clinic for next week)

1 mark current pregnancy Hx

- Started bleeding 4 hours ago. Began with spotting, but bleeding increasing to a steady trickle. No clots or products passed. Bleeding spontaneous, not post-coital

1 mark Hx of bleeding

- Lower abdominal cramps of increasing intensity started 2 hours ago

1 mark pain Hx

- Did have hyperemesis gravidarum up until 2 weeks ago. Minimal symptoms now

1 mark current pregnancy Sx

- Last had food/drink 6 hours ago
- Periods regular (bleeds 3 days, 28 days apart), not heavy or painful, no post-coital or intermenstrual bleeding. No vaginal discharge
- Was on oral contraceptive pill until 4 months ago. Never had an STD

- No past gynae history of note
1 mark Gynae Hx
- Last Pap smear 8 months ago, normal
½ mark Pap smear Hx
- No medical problems
- No past psych history
- Past surgical history: appendicectomy (open, uncomplicated) at 17 years old
- Lives with husband (good relationship); works in marketing; smokes 10 cigarettes/day; no alcohol or drugs
½ mark smoking/alcohol/drug Hx
- No allergies. Nil medications

Examination
- Visibly distressed patient
- Vitals: BP 120/60, PR 84, Temp 37°C, RR 12
1 mark for vitals
- Abdomen: old appendicectomy scar, no masses, generalised tenderness over lower abdomen
- Speculum: cervical os slightly open, fresh blood coming from the os, mild ectropion
- Bimanual Ex: 6/40 sized anteverted uterus, no palpable adnexal masses, mild generalised tenderness
1 mark for speculum/PV Ex of uterine size, os, adnexae

Investigations
- Pelvic ultrasound (vaginal)
- Blood group and antibodies
- FBE
- Quantitative βHCG
1 mark for U/S, ½ mark for blood group, ½ mark for βHCG

Q2
- Miscarriage (inevitable, incomplete or complete)
- Ectopic pregnancy
- Hydatidiform molar pregnancy (rare and unlikely)
- Bleeding from cervix or vagina, e.g. cervical ectropion (unlikely given examination findings of bleeding from os)
1 mark 'miscarriage' (only ½ if not specific type(s))
½ mark for each further diagnosis (to max of 1 mark)

Q3
- Need to check blood group. If rhesus negative and no antibodies give anti-D 250 IU.
1 mark
- IV access (group and hold optional, depending on bleeding – not needed in this case)

- Given ultrasound and βHCG results, patient has a non-viable intrauterine pregnancy

1 mark

Options for management
1 Suction curettage under general anaesthetic (counsel regarding risks: anaesthetic risks, retained products 1–2% requiring further treatment, infection, perforation of uterus <0.5%).
2 Medical treatment on ward with misoprostol 400 mcg PV 4/24ly until delivery of products.
3 Expectant management (given time, patient will likely pass pregnancy products on her own), with suction curette in case of excessive bleeding.

2 marks for all 3 options, 1 mark for 1–2 options

Q4
Counsel patient
Candidates should demonstrate appropriate sensitivity to patient's feelings by expressing some recognition of loss.

1 mark

- 15% of all pregnancies result in a miscarriage
- 25–50% of women will have at least one miscarriage in their lifetime
- 50–60% of all miscarriages due to sporadic chromosomal defects

½ mark

- No increased risk of miscarriage in the next pregnancy

½ mark

- Slight increased risk of miscarriage with smoking, can reduce risk by quitting

½ mark

- Needs folate 0.5 mg/day, and rubella status checked prior to next pregnancy

½ mark

- No increased risk of miscarriage risk from working, normal activity, sexual intercourse

½ mark

- No need for investigation for causes of miscarriage unless three consecutive miscarriages
- Refer to counselling services/support groups if necessary

½ mark
20 marks total

Discussion
'Miscarriage', or early pregnancy loss, is defined slightly differently in different countries. In Australia it is the loss of an intrauterine pregnancy at under 20 weeks gestation, or of a fetus weighing under 400 g where the gestation is not accurately known. In the UK it is under 24 weeks gestation, and the WHO defines a miscarriage as under 22 weeks, or under 500 g.

It is the most common pregnancy complication, affecting roughly 15% of all clinically recognised pregnancies, with risk increasing along with maternal age:

Maternal age (years)	Miscarriage risk
20–24	9%
25–29	11%
30–34	15%
35–39	25%
40–44	51%
45+	75%

In the 20 years between 1985 and 2004 the proportion of pregnant women in Victoria over 30 has almost doubled from 32.2% to 60%, and for women over 35 it has almost tripled from 7.8% to 22.4%, meaning that miscarriage rates are increasing. The increase in miscarriage rate related to maternal age is at least in part due to an increased risk of chromosomal aneuploidy in fetuses. The most common chromosomal abnormalities in miscarriages are trisomies (60%), monosomy X (Turner's syndrome) (15–25%), and triploidy (15–20%).

There are a number of risk factors for miscarriage apart from maternal age, including endocrine (poorly controlled diabetes, Graves' disease, hyperprolactinaemia), genetic (e.g. balanced reciprocal translocations in either parent), uterine structural abnormalities (submucosal fibroids, uterine septum, bicornuate uterus, cervical incompetence), infection (bacterial vaginosis, other pregnancy-related infections), antiphospholipid syndrome, and thrombophilias. None of them is relevant in this case, and should not be investigated for unless three consecutive miscarriages have occurred (defined as recurrent miscarriage, and found in only 1% of all couples). Other risk factors for miscarriage include chronic medical conditions, abdominal trauma, cigarette smoking, alcohol, cocaine use, and occupational/environmental exposure to various chemical agents (lead and organic solvents).

Mrs Turner is only 24 years old, and the only risk factor is her cigarette smoking. She should be encouraged to quit smoking, but candidates must be careful not to increase her feelings of guilt regarding the miscarriage. Smoking increases the risk of miscarriage, but it is still unlikely to be solely due to cigarette smoking.

The history and examination point to miscarriage as the most likely cause of the early pregnancy bleeding. Types of miscarriages are classified as in the table overleaf. Candidates should still be able to list the (unlikely) alternative diagnoses of ectopic pregnancy, hydatidiform molar pregnancy, and local cervical/vaginal causes. The past history of an appendicectomy does not increase the risk of an ectopic pregnancy. Only appendicectomy complicated by rupture and infection increases the ectopic risk.

	Symptoms	Cervical os	Ultrasound
Threatened miscarriage	Spotting Minimal pain	Closed	FH +ve
Inevitable miscarriage	Increased bleeding Cramping pains	Open	FH +ve
Incomplete miscarriage	Bleeding Pain variable	Open	FH-ve; some (? POC seen) POC still in uterus
Complete miscarriage	Reducing bleeding Pain variable	Closed	Uterus empty
Missed miscarriage	Nil or spotting	Closed	FH-ve
Septic miscarriage (can affect any of the above types)	Temperature Uterine tenderness	Variable	Variable

In relation to investigation and management, the blood group must be checked and anti-D immunoglobulin given to rhesus negative women, regardless of the cause of bleeding, to prevent isoimmunisation. The fetus has established a circulation and is producing red blood cells by about 5.5 weeks gestation. However, only the reduced dose of 250 IU is required for pregnancies under 14 weeks gestation. A pelvic ultrasound (with vaginal rather than abdominal scanning to provide more accurate information) is essential, both to pick up ectopic pregnancies (empty uterus or pseudosac, adnexal masses, free fluid in pelvis), hydatidiform molar pregnancies ('snow-storm' appearance of hydropic villi), as well as to aid in distinguishing between types of miscarriages, as seen above. If the pregnancy is non-viable, plans should be made to evacuate the uterus of pregnancy products by surgical, medical or expectant means.

The choice of evacuation method will be determined by a combination of the clinical condition of the patient, as well as by patient choice. For example, if haemodynamically compromised, a surgical option, being fastest, will be most appropriate. Be wary of using misoprostol for medical evacuation of a pregnancy in asthma sufferers, as misoprostol may cause bronchospasm. This is not an issue in the current patient, and any of the three options would be reasonable at the patient's discretion, given that she is medically stable.

The importance of a quantitative βHCG is in helping to interpret the ultrasound result. A fetal heart should be visible via vaginal ultrasound once the βHCG reaches 1500–2000 IU/mL; by abdominal ultrasound once it reaches 5000 IU/mL. During the first 10 weeks gestation in a viable pregnancy it should rise by at least 66% every 48 hours. In this case, with 8000 IU/mL, the pregnancy cannot be viable as a fetal heart is not visible by ultrasound. Another clue that the pregnancy has failed is the loss of early pregnancy symptoms (hyperemesis gravidarum) in the history.

When taking a history from the patient, focus on the presenting problem, but do not forget your general pregnancy management (e.g. ensuring the patient is on folate while trying to conceive to reduce the risk of neural tube defects, and checking rubella status).

In counselling the patient, the candidate should demonstrate sensitivity as a miscarriage is a distressing event. The risk of a miscarriage in a subsequent pregnancy increases with number of consecutive pregnancies roughly as follows:

After 1 miscarriage:	15% (unaltered)
2 miscarriages:	20% (slightly increased)
3 miscarriages:	30%
4 miscarriages:	40%
5 miscarriages:	50%

It is important to point out to the patient, even without her asking, that normal work, housework and sexual activity are not responsible for sporadic miscarriages. She may be feeling guilt about some of these, and she should be reassured. A miscarriage can cause a severe grief reaction similar to a stillbirth in some women, and they should be offered counselling and follow-up if necessary. There may be support groups available depending on the patient's location. Otherwise, her local doctor is a good start.

C3 Q1

History

- 30-year-old primigravida 38/40, singleton pregnancy
- No antenatal complications (no gestational diabetes or hypertension)
- Antenatal investigations including 20/40 ultrasound normal
- No history of fever/rash/illness
- No medical problems or past surgery
- NKA, nil medications, no alcohol/cigarettes/no illicit drug use
- Was working as office manager, and still working at diagnosis of FDIU
- Supportive, loving relationship with husband
- No fetal movements for 3 days prior to presentation

2 marks (depending on completeness)

Investigations

Explain to couple: Investigations are to look for a cause for the FDIU, so that the likelihood of recurrence and need for preventive measures in next pregnancy can be ascertained.

½ mark

Maternal investigations
- Blood group and antibodies (in case of isoimmunisation)
- FBE (if platelets low, may be disseminated intravascular coagulation (DIC))
- Fibrinogen
- APTT/INR
- Kleihauer test (if positive, may be concealed abruption)
- Serology screening for possible infections (toxoplasma, listeria, cytomegalovirus, rubella serology)
- HbA1C/glycosylated haemoglobin
- Thyroid function tests
- Antiphospholipid/anticardiolipin antibodies/lupus anticoagulant
- Antinuclear antigen (ANA)

2½ marks (½ for each point to maximum 2 ½)

Placenta/cord
- Send for histology after delivery
- Surface swabs for culture
- Examine cord for knots

1½ marks (½ for each point)

Fetal investigations (to be performed after delivery)
- Photographs for morphology assessment
- Karyotype (by skin biopsy)
- Surface swabs plus gastric aspirate for culture
- X-ray (particularly important if not consenting to autopsy)
- Autopsy: need to approach this with sensitivity and explain the need for an autopsy to determine if there are any issues found to explain the FDIU which may impact on future pregnancies. Must explain that it will only be performed with the permission of the parents, but that it is advisable to have one.

1 mark for discussion on autopsy
1½ marks (½ for each point to maximum of 1½ for the other points)

Q2

Some acknowledgement of the loss to the couple is appropriate, such as, "I am very sorry for the tragic loss of your baby."

2 marks for comment and appropriate manner

"There does not appear to be any cause based on the history, but we will need to wait for the results of the investigations we have ordered, and tests on the fetus after delivery." (or similar explanation)

½ mark

The fact that Mrs Harlow was working at the time had nothing to do with the stillbirth.

½ mark

Need to consider the options for delivery:
1 Would not advise a caesarean section, as this would create complications for future pregnancies/deliveries.
2 May opt for expectant management, as 80% of FDIUs will deliver spontaneously within 2 weeks. There is a risk of DIC, with slow consumption of fibrinogen over time, but the risk is low unless the FDIU remains in utero for >4 weeks.
3 Other option is for an induction of labour and vaginal delivery, using prostaglandins (low-dose misoprostol, or Prostin – prostaglandins E and F).

4 marks (1 for each point, and 1 for risk of DIC)

Before delivery, the couple needs to decide if they wish to see the stillborn baby or not. There is some evidence that seeing the baby after birth helps some couples to deal with the grieving process. Naming the baby is important to many couples, as well as having photos and neonatal footprints/handprints.

2 marks

Will need to consider options for burial of the stillborn baby at some stage.

½ mark

Will need to be offered counselling, and referral to support groups, such as SANDS (Stillbirth and Neonatal Death Support).

1 mark

Should see a senior consultant within 2 weeks after delivery of the stillbirth to go through the results of the investigations and autopsy, and plan for any special measures needed in subsequent pregnancies.

½ mark
20 marks maximum

Discussion

Tragically, up to half of all fetal deaths in utero occur at term. When they occur the couple require intense counselling and support. However, the practitioner must not lose sight of trying to find the cause of the FDIU so that the risk to subsequent pregnancies, if any, can be determined, and efforts can be made to prevent a recurrence. Unfortunately, many FDIUs at term remain unexplained, which can make it difficult for the couple to come to terms with the loss.

In subsequent pregnancies, with an unexplained term FDIU, the couple may require greater support and more frequent antenatal visits. While excessive fetal monitoring should not be encouraged for these patients, they may need reassurance that their baby is well, particularly when nearing the gestation at which they lost their previous baby. Delivery may need to be arranged by induction of labour or caesarean section (as the patient directs) at a gestation just prior to the previous loss, and if in labour, continuous fetal monitoring may be offered for parental reassurance in some centres.

All maternity units should have a protocol for managing and investigating FDIUs, so that staff do not fail to obtain potentially valuable information for the unfortunate parents.

C4 The student is expected to take an adequate history of the presenting problem and advise regarding surgical termination of pregnancy and post-procedure contraception.

Q1
History
- 24 years old
- First pregnancy
- Currently sexually active with 1 partner. Same partner for the last 2 years but relationship broke up when the pregnancy was diagnosed
- Usually uses condoms but not always compliant. Has used the combined oral contraceptive pill (COCP) in past but has had problems remembering to take it
- Periods generally occur every 28 days, lasting 5 days with no problems. LMP 10 weeks ago. Pregnancy dating confirmed on ultrasound as being 10 weeks gestation
- No past history – medical or surgical
- No family history
- No allergies, no medications, non-smoker, occasional alcohol
- Pap smear normal 12 months ago
- Requesting a TOP as feels unable to cope psychologically with a pregnancy on her own. Her parents live interstate. Has thought about the implications for her of having a TOP. Was initially shocked that she was pregnant but now resigned to the TOP as she feels it is the best decision for her
- Works as a secretary

8 marks maximum, depending on completeness of history

Q2
- Would be a surgical TOP due to gestation
- Suction currette under general anaesthetic or sedation. Short procedure with an oxytocic used to contract the uterus during the procedure
- Cervical preparation using 400 µg misoprostol vaginally at least 3 hours beforehand
- Doxycycline 100 mg orally 6 hours prior to procedure and 200 mg orally 2 hours after the procedure
- Must know blood group if have to administer Anti D

4 marks

Risks
- Perforation, which is minimised by the use of misoprostol, allowing gentle cervical dilatation

- Haemorrhage, which is minimised by the use of misoprostol and an oxytocic which contract the uterus
- Infection, which is minimised by the use of antibiotics
- No long-term sequelae

4 marks (1 for each point)

Q3
- Need to have adequate ongoing contraception so that not faced with an unplanned pregnancy again
- Reliable options include hormonal contraception such as Implanon, Depo-Provera, Mirena IUD or non-hormonal such as copper IUD. These forms of contraception can be administered at the time of a TOP
- All forms must be combined with the use of condoms with casual sexual partners

4 marks
20 marks total

Background information on termination of pregnancy
Abortion is not unlawful in the state of Victoria, provided that the medical practitioner can prove the health (mental or physical) of the mother would be endangered by continuing with the pregnancy. Abortion laws vary between states in Australia. In Victoria one abortion is performed for every three live births.

The annual worldwide abortion rate varies between 32 and 46 per 1,000 women aged 15–44 years, with a peak rate at the age of 20 years. In most developed countries the abortion rate varies between 10 and 30 per 1,000 women. Some 24% of the world's population reside in countries where abortion is not legally permitted. Worldwide about 2 out of 5 abortions are thought to be illegal, leading to between 50,000 to 100,000 preventable deaths each year, nearly all (99%) in poor countries. Each hour 8 women die from unsafe abortions.

There is evidence that improving sex education and particularly promoting access to safe and effective contraception decreases the number of abortions performed in any country. Abortion is ultimately a choice that the individual woman makes with or without consultation with the father, members of her family, a religious advisor or her doctor.

The number of abortions performed in order to protect the physical health of the mother is few. Termination of pregnancy is also indicated if the mother has ingested a potential teratogen during the period of organogenesis, or if the fetus is known to have an abnormality. Less than 2% of abortions are for fetal abnormality.

Psychological or social indications comprise the major reason for the performance of pregnancy termination in this country. Most abortions are induced because the pregnancy is unintended and unwanted. A minority of women request abortion because of a psychiatric illness severe enough to require intervention. However, an unwanted or accidental pregnancy can cause severe psychological stress.

Counselling is a most important part of the management of a woman who requests pregnancy termination. The major objectives of counselling are:

• to determine the reason for pregnancy termination
• to discuss the implications of the request
• to offer emotional support
• to discuss future contraceptive options.

First trimester abortion

The risk of **surgical abortion** is reduced if it is performed in the first trimester. This procedure ranks among the safest and easiest surgical procedures with a mortality rate of 1/100,000 procedures. In developed countries the mortality associated with childbirth is 11 times higher than that associated with safely performed surgical abortion and 30 times higher than for abortions performed up to 8 weeks gestation. More than 90% of terminations are performed in the first trimester of pregnancy. The most common surgical procedure is vacuum aspiration (98%), which can take place until 14 weeks gestation. All procedures are performed under local (paracervical block) or general anaesthesia. Pre-operative cervical preparation should be undertaken. The optimal drug is misoprostol and the optimal dosage and time interval of misoprostol appears to be 400 µg vaginally 3 h prior to the termination (grade A evidence). The cervix should be dilated as atraumatically as possible and as little as is necessary to perform the operation safely. After cervical dilatation, an oxytocic drug (0.5 mg ergometrine intravenously [IV] or 10IU syntocinon IV) is administered and the suction currettage performed under a vacuum pressure of 800 mmHg. If there is doubt as to whether the uterus is empty, the cavity can be explored using a sharp currette. An empty uterus usually does *not* bleed. Surgical termination should not be performed at ≤6 weeks gestation due to failure to remove the gestational sac, but medical abortion (see below) is most effective at ≤7 weeks gestation. After the procedure the products of conception are routinely sent for histological assessment.

Medical abortion is the method of choice at ≤7 weeks and should be offered at 7–9 weeks gestation. It is a safe and effective procedure. This method of pregnancy termination can be accomplished using 200 mg RU486 with 800 µg Misoprostol administered vaginally 48 h later (grade A evidence). The addition of the latter reduces the dose of each individual medication and reduces the side effects, which are mainly gastrointestinal. When the drugs are given in combination, 5% require a currettage, 1% will bleed heavily enough to require a transfusion and the method will fail in 1%. The abortion usually occurs within 6 h of the administration of the PG analogue in 90% and within 8 h in 96%.

Routine follow-up is mandatory if this method of pregnancy termination is used. The success rate depends on the length of the pregnancy and if performed early has a success rate similar to vacuum aspiration. A Cochrane review has reported that medical methods of abortion in early pregnancy are safe and effective, with the best evidence for the combination of RU486 and misprostol. As yet there are no currently available studies directly comparing surgical termination of pregnancy with this combination of medications.

Second trimester abortion

In the **second trimester surgical abortion** involves dilatation and evacuation (D&E) with misoprostol 400 μg 3-hourly for 3 doses administered vaginally beforehand. This method of surgical abortion is cheaper and safer than medical methods. It is performed under intubational anaesthesia after 14–16 weeks gestation and volatile anaesthetic gases must not be used. Serious complications occur in 1% and include perforation, cervical damage and retained products.

A **medical termination in the second trimester** can be carried out using vaginal (PGE_1 or PGE_2), intramniotic or intramuscular PGs. Extra or intraamniotic PGE_2 compares well in terms of efficacy with D&E. PGE_1 pessaries, such as misoprostol 400 μg can also be placed in the posterior fornix of the vagina every 3–4 h, with 5–6 being required to cause an abortion.

The most important determinants of abortion **mortality** are gestation at the time of the procedure and the type of anaesthesia used. **Early complications** of first trimester surgical abortion include uterine perforation, haemorrhage, cervical lacerations, failure to complete the procedure due to performance too early in gestation and anaesthetic mishaps. **Late complications** include retained products (0.2–0.6%), anaemia, thromboembolism and cervical stenosis (0.02%). The mortality rate is 1:100,000 from infection (23%), thromboembolism (23%), haemorrhage (20%) and anaesthesia (16%).

Pelvic infection may complicate up to 12% of surgically induced abortions. A meta-analysis of randomised trials showed that prophylaxis with antibiotics effective against either *Chlamydia trachomatis* or *bacterial vaginosis* reduced the post-abortion infective morbidity by half. The screen and treat strategy appears to be less cost-effective than routine prophylaxis.

The perforation rate in first trimester surgical terminations is 0.05% and in second trimester procedures is 0.32%. Perforation may occur at the cervical-uterine junction during dilatation or during the curettage. The suction curette may then be placed behind the bladder or in front of the rectum. During the procedure most perforations occur at the fundus and usually go unrecognised. If a perforation is suspected the extent of the damage must be assessed. If there is no active bleeding, no action is necessary. However, if the defect is large, there is active bleeding or there is a suspicion of bowel injury, laparoscopy +/– laparotomy must be performed. If a perforation does occur the procedure may be completed under laparoscopic or ultrasound guidance, or alternatively may be performed, 2 weeks later. Risk factors for perforation are previous gynaecological surgery including previous abortion, lower uterine segment caesarian section and large loop excision of the transformation zone of the cervix. Atraumatic pre-operative dilation of the cervix using PGs may prevent this important complication.

Vacuum aspiration in the first trimester is not associated with later infertility, increased risk of ectopic pregnancy or subsequent non-viable outcome. First trimester abortion is also not associated with later spontaneous miscarriage. There is also no association with an increased risk of breast cancer. It is uncertain if second trimester abortions ultimately affect fertility.

Studies have shown that the **psychological sequelae** of abortion are minimal for the majority of women and that choosing to terminate a pregnancy rather than deliver an unwanted first pregnancy does not place women at higher risk of depression. Indeed, the prevention of abortion may be psychologically more devastating for the woman and her child. After pregnancy termination most women express relief. Feelings of guilt and loss are usually self-limiting. The women who may have difficulty coping with an abortion are those who are:

- dependent on alcohol or drugs or who live in an abusive relationship and have poor social supports
- victims of rape or incest
- aborting because of fetal abnormality or at an advanced gestational age at the time of the termination
- suffering from a pre-existing psychiatric illness
- unsure about going ahead with an abortion.

In Rh negative women, anti-D prophylaxis must not be forgotten.

C5 Q1

N.B. This OSCE station is best examined with a doll for the candidate to demonstrate the resuscitation steps on. A stethoscope and neonatal resuscitation mask are helpful, if available, but not essential (the candidate can indicate that they use them whether or not they are present by miming the necessary actions).

At birth, should immediately assess if baby is breathing, crying, and whether or not there is good tone.

1 mark

EXAMINER: "The baby is not breathing, and has no muscular tone."

- Should dry and provide tactile stimulation to the baby (e.g. with towel/cloth/rubbing of skin)
- Provide warmth to the baby (radiant heat source)
- Position the airway – head should be in neutral or slightly extended position (if overextended, may block airway)
- Check breathing, and check heart rate with stethoscope

4 marks (1 mark for each)

EXAMINER: "The baby is still not breathing and has a heart rate of about 80 beats/minute."
● Need to initiate positive pressure ventilation, using air or oxygen, either with self-inflating bag or a T-piece resuscitation device (e.g. Neopuff). The latter provides PEEP (positive end expiratory pressure) and ventilations should be administered at a rate of 60 times per minute.

2 marks

● Reassess every minute or so for attempts by infant at respiration, as well as heart rate auscultation.

1 mark

EXAMINER: "The baby is still not breathing, and the heart rate has dropped to 40 beats/minute."
● Commence chest compressions: Place hands around the chest with two thumbs over the lower half of the baby's sternum (1 finger's breadth below a line drawn between the nipples), compressing the thumbs down on the sternum so that one-third of the chest anterior-posterior diameter is depressed.
● Should perform 90 chest compressions and 30 ventilations in 1 minute, with a ratio of 3:1.

3 marks

● Reassess the respiratory efforts, heart rate, colour and tone of the baby regularly.

1 mark

EXAMINER: "The baby starts to cry after 3 minutes of resuscitation, the heart rate has increased to 120 beats/minute, and the baby is now pink with good tone."
● Cease resuscitation, keep baby warm.

1 mark

Q2
The Apgar score is from 0 to 10, and is used to identify infants in need of resuscitation. Apgar scores are routinely determined and recorded at 1 minute and 5 minutes after birth. They are determined by a score between 0 and 2 for each of the following five signs:

Sign	Score = 0	Score = 1	Score = 2
Heart rate	Absent	<100 bpm	>100 bpm
Respiration	Absent	Weak/irregular	Regular/crying
Colour	White/blue	Pale extremities Body pink	Completely pink
Tone	Flaccid	Reduced	Well flexed
Irritability/Reflexes	None	Reduced	Cough/cry

2 marks for why Apgars performed
5 marks for each criterion for Apgar (1 mark each)
20 marks total

Discussion

A knowledge of basic neonatal resuscitation is expected to be demonstrated by the examination candidate in this station. The resuscitation described is based on the guidelines of the Australian Resuscitation Council.

The flowchart on the opposite page can be obtained from the website: http://www.resus.org.au/arc_neonatal_flowchart.pdf

C6

In the OSCE exam, there would be a mannequin for the student to demonstrate the performance of a Pap smear on. In this practice OSCE the exam candidate should mime the actions of the Pap smear, or describe the steps verbally.

The student is expected to go through the process of performing a Pap smear on the mannequin. They are expected to understand the different steps in the performance of a Pap smear and to understand why these tests are performed and how frequently they should occur.

Equipment required

- Mannequin
- Bivalve speculum
- Cytobrush or cervex brush
- Wooden spatula
- Fixative
- Lubricant or water
- Glass slides
- Slide covers
- Pencil
- Adequate lighting

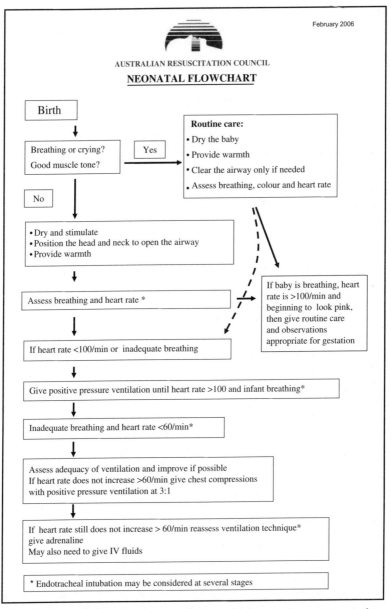

Figure 4.2 The assessment for resuscitation and subsequent management of a newborn baby in the absence of meconium

Q1

The student is expected to state that Pap smears are performed to detect pre-cancerous cervical changes or cervical dysplasia. It is a screening test that shows there may be changes, but does not give a definite diagnosis of what the changes are. If there is an abnormal result the patient should be referred for a colposcopy (examination of the cervix with a bifocal microscope by a gynaecologist). Pap smears are done every 2 years in the absence of problems.

4 marks total, depending on completeness of the answer

Q2

The student is expected to go through the process of:
1 writing detail on the slide
2 getting the equipment necessary, such as speculum, brush and spatula, fixative and slide cover
3 warming the speculum with water
4 inserting the speculum into the vagina and displaying the cervix and fixing the speculum
5 with the spatula, rotating the pointy end 360° in the internal os to sample the transformation zone
6 with the cytobrush or cervex brush, rotating it 360° in the internal os to sample the transformation zone
7 fixation of the slide and placing in the slide holder
8 removal of the speculum.

16 marks (2 marks for each point)

Discussion

Pap smears (named after Papanicolaou, the inventor of the test) are performed as a screening test to identify cervical dysplasia before it progresses to cervical carcinoma. The Pap smear is an example of 'exfoliative cytology'. It is not a diagnostic test. The smear samples cells from the 'transformation zone' of the cervix. The transformation zone is the point of transition from columnar to squamous epithelium and is the site at which squamous cell cervical carcinomas are most likely to occur. The cells are preserved on a slide for examination. The proportion of cells on the slide with abnormal characteristics, such as poor differentiation, increased nuclear-cytoplasm ratio, hyperchromasia, and nuclear pleomorphism, determines whether the smear is described as CIN I-III or mild to severe dysplasia. Because the Pap smear is a screen, in the case of abnormality all women with an abnormal Pap smear should have a colposcopy. A colposcopy enables a targeted biopsy of the abnormal area to occur, thus giving a definitive diagnosis of the degree of the abnormality. The woman can then be appropriately treated prior to the development of a cancer.

In Australia it is recommended for women every 2 years until 70 years of age, starting one year after the first episode of sexual intercourse. The reason that the incidence of cervical cancer has decreased is due to the performance of Pap smears. In Australia, women who present with cervical cancers tend to be those who have never had a Pap smear.

Pre-cancerous lesions of the cervix are associated with infection with oncogenic strains of the human papilloma virus (HPV). A prophylactic HPV vaccine is now available in Australia and New Zealand to prevent infection with some of the more common oncogenic strains of HPV. RANZCOG recommends the vaccination of all females aged 9 to 26 years against HPV. It is expected that this will reduce the incidence of cervical dysplasia in the future. However, despite vaccination, current recommended screening protocols should continue to be adhered to.

C7 Q1
History
- Take a history for any medical conditions, allergies and medications to ensure there are no contra-indications to any methods of analgesia
- Medical Hx: childhood asthma now resolved
- Surgical Hx: appendicectomy
- Family Hx: nil significant
- Medications: Blackmores multivitamins for pregnancy and breastfeeding
- Allergies: penicillin – rash

½ mark each (maximum 1 mark)

Discuss the patient's options, commencing with drug-free methods, then moving on to prescribed analgesia and then anaesthesia.

1 Drug-free methods: mobilising – walking, rocking; position change – bean bag, floor mat, mediball; hot packs; massage; water-based shower, bath

½ mark each (maximum 1 mark)

2 Patient-controlled analgesia: nitrous oxide, TENS

½ mark each (maximum 1 mark)

3 Prescribed analgesia: oral, IM, IV: Panadol/Panadeine/Panadeine forte, IM pethidine (uncommon: IV pethidine)

½ mark each (maximum 1 mark)

4 Anaesthesia: epidural block, spinal block, combined epidural/spinal

½ mark each (maximum 1 mark)

5 marks total

Q2
1 Drug-free methods
Advantages
- No medications
- No needles or injections
- No risk of fetal or maternal sedation
- Multiple options
- Patient remains in control
- Partner can be involved

1 mark each (3 marks maximum)

Disadvantages
- May not be adequate for some women's analgesia needs
- Water-based therapy cannot be used with continuous CTG monitoring
- Movement options may be limited if continuous monitoring is required

½ mark for any one of the above

2 Patient-controlled analgesia
Nitrous oxide
Advantages
- Rapid onset/rapid offset
- Can be used for many hours
- Patient-controlled
- No overdose/sedation risk
- Provides a reasonable level of analgesia

1 mark each (3 marks maximum)

Disadvantages
- Nausea
- Dry mouth
- Dizziness
- Mask can be claustrophobic
- May not be adequate for some women's needs

½ mark each (1 mark maximum)

TENS
Advantages
- No sedation
- No nausea

½ mark for any one of the above

Disadvantages
- Limited analgesic benefit
- Cannot use water-based therapy

½ mark for any one of the above

3 Prescribed analgesia
Advantages
- Provides reasonable analgesia
- Routinely available
- Does not require IV access

½ mark each (1 mark maximum)

Disadvantages
- Nausea/vomiting
- Maternal: altered conscious state/sedation
- Fetal sedation/ respiratory compromise
- local pain/hematoma at injection site
- Rare risk of nerve damage (sciatic nerve)
- Intermittent administration is required

- Not appropriate analgesia for heroin-using clients

1 mark each (2 marks maximum)

4 Anaesthesia
Advantages
- Usually provides excellent pain relief

½ mark

Disadvantages
- Requires specialised operator (anaesthetist)
- Rare risk of complications: abscess, hematoma, nerve injury
- Risk of failure, incomplete block
- Requires IV access, CTG monitoring, in-dwelling catheter
- Loss of mobility due to motor blockade
- Possible maternal hypotension
- Post-dural puncture headache
- Increased requirement for Syntocinon augmentation
- May be contra-indicated for some congenital or acquired spinal disease and some medical illnesses e.g. lumbar disc disease, multiple sclerosis

½ mark each (3 marks maximum)

15 marks total (Q2)

20 marks total

Discussion

Overview
As with any clinical encounter, the student is expected to briefly review the relevant clinical history at the commencement of the OSCE. Although it would be uncommon to find according to the antenatal history that any particular method of pain relief is contra-indicated, this still demonstrates that the candidate shows a logical and clinically oriented approach to the problem. The candidate is then expected to show a sensible progression to the answer, beginning with widely available, low-tech, low-risk pain relief options and working through to the most effective but least available and most interventional methods of pain relief.

Discussion
The experience and implications of labour pain varies widely between women and may even vary between labours for the same woman. Pain is commonly experienced as lower abdominal pain during contractions that can extend to intermittent or continuous lumbo-sacral back pain, and gluteal or thigh pain. Pain has been variably reported as up to horrible or excruciating. On average, labour pain increases with progressive cervical dilatation and depends upon the intensity, duration and frequency of uterine contractions. As normal labour still represents a physiological phenomenon, researchers are still divided as to whether labour pain has significant detrimental effects. The potential negative physiological effects of labour pain include increased cardiac output, increased blood pressure and heart rate and hyperventilation.

Intra-partum pain relief options vary widely depending upon ethnic origin, cultural practices, location of birth and individual expectations. Continuous trained labour support, including both emotional and physical assistance, has been demonstrated to reduce the usage of intra-partum analgesia, increase the likelihood of a spontaneous vaginal birth, increase the woman's satisfaction with the birth experience, and has no known risks. This is of greatest benefit when begun early in labour.

Bathing during labour is safe and appears to be most effective when used beyond 5 cm dilatation for limited periods. Bath use may be of benefit by increasing maternal relaxation and decreasing catecholamine production. Bathing temperature should be kept to 36–37°C to prevent maternal hyperthermia and potential neonatal morbidity. Studies are divided upon the overall effectiveness of bathing during labour for pain relief.

Studies of the benefits of positioning in labour for pain relief are limited and difficult to conduct. However, the freedom to adopt the position of choice considered most beneficial by the mother for reduction of pain should be encouraged.

Nitrous oxide inhaled via an on-demand valve is widely used in Australia. It can be used at any stage of labour, for any duration of time and is widely accepted due to its ease of use, minimal side-effects, and absence of effect on uterine activity. Due to the intermittent nature of uterine contraction-related pain and the time lag between the commencement of inhalation and the onset of analgesic effect, nitrous oxide is most effective if inhaled before the commencement of the contraction, but in practice this can be difficult to achieve. Quantitative effects of nitrous oxide on pain scores have been difficult to validate scientifically; however, in many studies, labouring women describe significant analgesic effect with nitrous oxide use.

A **TENS** (transcutaneous electrical nerve stimulation) consists of a stimulator and a pair of electrodes. The stimulator contains a pulse generator and two controls for amplitude, for amplitude and frequency. It is attached to the spinal processes of the patient, and impulses cause muscle fasciculation to alter the sensation of pain during uterine contractions. It is a non-invasive option of pain relief, but while effective for some women, does not have as strong an analgesic effect as more invasive options discussed below.

Epidural anaesthesia is a nerve block technique using local anaesthetic and/or opioid agents that requires the skills of a specialist anaesthetist. Side effects such as pruritis, nausea, vomiting, inability to void, impaired motor blockade, an increased likelihood of instrumental delivery, a greater need for oxytocin augmentation, and risks of maternal hypotension and fever are all well recognised. A lumbar epidural technique is the most widely used, but combined spinal/epidural (CSE) approaches are also possible. A CSE offers the spinal advantages of faster onset of analgesic effect, with the epidural advantages of continuous infusion and ongoing analgesia. In general, an epidural anaesthesia is more effective for labour pain relief than non-epidural methods but it has more side effects and complications. Minor side effects such as pruritis and nausea depend upon the inclusion of opioid in the epidural agents. Pruritis rates for local anaesthetic agents alone range from 0–4%, but up to an average of 62% in the presence of narcotic agents. Nausea and vomiting rates overall are low, on average <5%. At least 60% of women require an indwelling catheter for an inability to void spontaneously and in many centres the use of an indwelling catheter is routine with epidural usage to avoid the risks of urinary retention and bladder overdistension. Hypotension rates are variable and can occur in up to 50% of labouring women following epidural insertion. Prophylactic intravenous fluid administration may be of benefit. According to the Cochrane collaboration, epidural anaesthesia increases the risk of instrumental delivery (RR1.38), maternal fever >38 °C (RR 3.6) with no demonstrated effect upon caesarean section rates, neonatal Apgar scores or long-term backache.

C8 Encounter 1
History
- Mrs W, 62 years old
- Currently fit and well. Had surgery 3 months ago for endometrial cancer (surgical cure, with no further treatment required)
- G6P6 (3 daughters, 3 sons, all NVDs)
- Past Hx: R Breast cancer (aged 52; treated with wide local excision and axillary clearance. Had tamoxifen for 2 years, then arimidex, as developed an endometrial polyp with tamoxifen)
- Non-drinker, non-smoker
- NKA meds – Arimidex
- Family Hx:
  – Daughter died of bowel cancer aged 30
  – All 5 other children have had colonic polyps removed, and have regular colonoscopies for screening
  – Father died of bowel cancer aged 76
  – Mother alive and well
  – No other siblings
  – History for grandparents unknown
- Lives in rural area; runs a dairy farm with her husband, one son, and his family; other children live in the nearest city; 6 grandchildren

9 marks

Encounter 2
- Strong family history of bowel cancer (2 first-degree relatives: father and daughter). Also personal history of breast and endometrial cancer
- Recommend review at a familial cancer clinic for consideration of genetic testing

3 marks

Encounter 3
- Hereditary non-polyposis colorectal cancer (HNPCC)
- Hereditary breast and ovarian cancer (BRCA1 and BRCA2)

2 marks

Encounter 4
- HNPCC – colonoscopy for bowel cancer/no screening test for endometrial cancer
  – colectomy
- BRCA 1/2 – mammography (breast), CA125 + pelvic U/S (ovary)
  – prophylactic mastectomies (breast), prophylactic BSO (ovary)

6 marks

20 marks total

Discussion
The medical student is expected to display a basic understanding of some common hereditary cancer syndromes. The patient has a strong family history of bowel cancer, as well as a personal history of endometrial and breast cancer. Hereditary non-polyposis colorectal cancer should be suspected, and the patient referred to an appropriate genetic cancer counselling service. While the students are not expected to counsel the patient as to options for prophylactic treatment (i.e. whether or not to have a prophylactic colectomy), they are expected to be aware of the known options for screening or prophylactic surgery in these cases.

STUDENT OSCE D

D1 Q1
N.B. obstetric emergency, so need to keep history-taking brief
- Medical history? Nil
- Surgical history? Nil
- Family history? Nil
- Medications? Nil
- Allergies? Nil
- Pap smear: at first visit, normal result obtained
- Progress of the pregnancy to date: any complications such as gestational hypertension, gestational diabetes? No

Presenting complaint
- Bleeding: approx 0100. Woken from sleep; found self lying in a pool of blood on bed. Went to toilet, more fresh bleeding into the bowl. Called the ambulance.
- Amount: at least 2 cups
- Site: vaginal
- Appearance: fresh, bright, like blood from a cut finger

Associated features
- Pain: nil initially, now some crampy period pains

- ROM: not noted
- Uterine activity period pains as noted
- Fetal movements present

No ROM
Pain
Fetal movements
No significant medical surgical history
No allergies
3 marks (1 mark each, any 3 of above)

Q2
- BP 115/70
- HR 100
- Periphery warm and well perfused

BP
HR
Peripheries
2 marks (1 point each any 2)

Abdo:
- symphysiofundal height = 34 weeks
- uterine tenderness = moderate
- lie: longitudinal
- presentation: cephalic, mobile
- presence of fetal heart: detected
- Timing-tightenings, 2 in 10
- Bleeding: fresh blood on pads, soaking approx 1 pad every 20 mins

Tenderness
Uterine activity
Fetal lie/presentation
Fetal heart
4 marks (1 each)

- Speculum Ex: Clot present
- Total measured loss from clots = 100 mL
- Active fresh bleeding seen through os
- Exclude local lower genital tract causes of bleeding– nil sites seen

Bleeding
Ongoing loss
Speculum examination: Exclude lower causes
Identify blood through os
3 marks

Q3
- IV bung

- IV fluids– colloid/crystalloid to replace loss at least 600 mL

Resuscitation/maternal stabilization
IV bung
IV colloid/crystalloid
3 marks

- X- match blood (2 units)
- Kleihauer
- APPT/INR or clotting studies

2 marks (any 2 of above: 1 mark each)

- Continuous CTG monitoring while bleeding

1 mark

- Fast while actively bleeding
- Notify registrar/specialist/senior member of staff
- Prepare for delivery if fetal distress or ongoing haemorrhage
- Urgent ultrasound for placental site

1 mark (½ mark each for any of the above)

Q4

- Placental abruption

1 mark
20 marks total

Discussion

This is a difficult station for the medical student as it requires the student to simultaneously consider directed history-taking, specific points on examination, as well as basic steps of resuscitation and management in a time-pressured setting. As such, it helps to differentiate the student who has spent time in the delivery suite and seen how such cases are managed in this way in a real-life setting, where history, examination and management are frequently combined in similar urgent scenarios. This ability to manage multiple threads of information only comes with practice. In this scenario, designed to simulate a major, evolving abruptio placenta, the history required is brief and directed towards major life-threatening issues that would interfere with surgery or an anaesthetic.

Basic minimums that must be obtained in such a scenario include: any prior operations or anaesthetics? Any major medical illnesses/chronic conditions, e.g. asthma, diabetes, hypertension? Any medications or drugs of dependence? Any allergies? Every doctor should have a standard list of major questions to ask in any emergency setting and this is a good time to practise using it even if the introduction has stated that the patient was previously well. In this setting, asking for a handheld record from the patient can be of immense benefit, but may not be available.

Once the basic history has been obtained the examination needs to be directed towards the immediate wellbeing of the mother and the fetus, as well as the cause of the bleeding, with the background plan of whether the fetus requires immediate or semi-urgent delivery within the next 24 hours.

It is easy to forget that a young, fit woman may have lost significant blood volume before there are any physiological signs of compromise; conversely, anxiety may induce a tachycardia that is out of sync with the other physical signs. Typically, a blood loss of 15% of total circulating volume will have no effect on measured heart rate or blood pressure, and the patient will still have warm, well-perfused peripheries. Signs of mild shock may not be evident until a blood loss of 20–25%, progressing to profound hypotension and collapse once the blood loss reaches 40% of circulating volume. Even if a non-invasive monitor is used to regularly record the blood pressure and heart rate, laying hands on the patient's pulse still provides invaluable information about the quality of the pulse and the peripheries, and is to be encouraged in all emergency situations.

The examination then progresses to an assessment of the abdomen and the gravid uterus, looking both for clues as to the cause of bleeding and clinical information that may impact upon the management of the pregnancy. The two most common causes of APH are abruptio and placenta praevia, and the history has already indicated that the 20-week ultrasound showed a non-praevia placenta. This is reassuring at approximately 99% accuracy, so it is rare but not impossible to find a missed placenta praevia or succenturiate lobe not recognised at the 20-week scan.

D2 Encounter 1
History
- Mrs D, 62 years old
- Has had a 'lump' in the vagina for several years. Associated with a dragging sensation. Become much worse over the last 3–4 months
- Sometimes has to push the lump back in order to empty her bowels
- Urinary incontinence slowly worsening over the last few years
- Loses urine when laughs, coughs, sneezes, jumps, losing small amounts of urine; needs to wear an incontinence pad all the time during the day 'just in case'; has 3–4 episodes of incontinence per week
- Goes to the toilet 8 times per day ("to keep my bladder empty and prevent accidents"), and gets up once in the night
- Occasional urgency, but not the major feature of the incontinence. No double-voiding
- No incontinence of flatus or faeces. No constipation; normal bowel habit
- Not sexually active (husband has Alzheimer's)
- Drinks 4 cups of coffee per day, and has a couple of glasses of wine in the evenings
- Has had 6 normal vaginal deliveries of 7 children (one set of twins born vaginally); had 'quick labours'
- Menopausal at 50 years old, no post-menopausal bleeding; used hormone therapy for 5 years for hot flushes, then stopped due to concern regarding her breast cancer risk
- Last Pap smear 15 years ago (normal)

- Never had a mammogram
- Past medical Hx: hypertension (Rx atenolol; well-controlled)
- Past surgery: open cholecystectomy (10 years ago); bilateral total knee joint replacement (5 years ago); appendicectomy aged 10 y.o.
- No allergies; meds: atenolol
- Lives with husband (Alzheimer's), and also looks after her severely disabled grand-daughter (cerebral palsy) 5 days a week while her daughter works. Her daughter is reliant on this help
- Ex-smoker (quit 12 years ago); drinks wine (2 glasses) in the evening

Encounter 2
Examination
- Obese woman, BMI 38
- BP 135/90, PR 72, T 37 C, RR 16
- Chest clear, No breast lumps
- Abdomen: moderate pannus, no masses
- Vulva: normal
- Sims speculum Ex: Grade 4 uterine descent (procidentia), Grade 2 rectocele, Grade 2 cystocele; cervix has some ulceration, with a dry and wrinkled appearance (can perform Pap smear); Stress incontinence demonstrated after reduction of the uterus

Encounter 3
Issues include:
1 the severe utero-vaginal prolapse
2 the urinary incontinence
3 general health issues.
Investigations required include:
- mid-stream urine for culture, to rule out a bladder infection
- urodynamics studies to determine if the major cause of urinary incontinence is stress or urge (N.B. will need to perform studies with uterus replaced into the pelvis, or the procidentia may mask more severe stress incontinence)
- ECG, CXR (hypertension and risk of heart disease from obesity), to determine suitability/risk of surgery.
Prolapse quite severe, and pelvic floor exercises are unlikely to be of assistance.

Options for treatment include insertion of a ring pessary or surgery (vaginal hysterectomy, anterior and posterior vaginal repair combined with a type of vault suspension procedure). If opting for surgery, will need to arrange assistance for care of her husband and grand-daughter, and will need medical review.

If, as appears likely, the urinary incontinence is mainly stress incontinence, surgery for prolapse can be combined with a sling/mesh procedure such as a TVT (tension-free vaginal tape) or Monarc sling.

In general, she should reduce her coffee and alcohol intake to improve her bladder control.

Obesity is a general health issue: should be encouraged to lose weight (diet/exercise).

She needs to have a mammogram every 2 years for screening.

She should probably should have a diabetes screen (glucose tolerance test) and fasting cholesterol/triglycerides (at risk due to obesity).

(Mrs D's urodynamics confirms severe stress incontinence, and she decides on a ring pessary as well as a TVT procedure.)

Discussion
In this case, the student is expected to demonstrate the ability to take an appropriate history and perform the appropriate examination for urinary incontinence. As in this case, there is often a range of health issues facing such patients, and it is important to deal with all of the appropriate health issues – not just the prolapse and incontinence.

When deciding on treatment options, the candidate must consider the social context. In this case, a ring pessary, combined with a day procedure such as a TVT sling procedure may be more appealing to the patient than a major operation, given the dependence of her husband and grand-daughter. A good candidate will consider the social situation in their counselling of the patient. It must be noted that a ring pessary is inappropriate if the patient is sexually active.

A urine culture is mandatory before considering treatment for urinary incontinence, as a urine infection may masquerade as stress or urge incontinence, triggering unnecessary surgery or medical treatment.

D3 Q1
History
- Mrs Walker, 25-year-old G1P0 39/40 gestation
- Singleton pregnancy
- No antenatal problems (no gestational diabetes or hypertension)
- Blood group A positive
- No medical problems; no past Hx surgery
- No allergies. Nil medications
- Had a show 8 hours ago; membranes intact
- Started contracting 6 hours ago, with frequency of contractions increasing from 10-minutely to 5-minutely contractions 3 hours ago
- Fetal movements felt today; fetal heart heard with intermittent auscultation (fetal heart rate 140–150 bpm)
- Using nitrous oxide gas for analgesia, and coping well

4 marks, depending on completeness

Examination
- BP 120/80, PR 92, T 37°C
- Abdominal Ex: fundus = dates (term), longitudinal lie, cephalic presentation, 4/5 of head palpable above the pelvic brim, fetal heart rate 150 bpm with doppler
- 2 in 10 moderate contractions

2 marks

- Vaginal Ex (with patient's permission):
  - Cervix 4 cm dilated, 1 cm long, and in mid-position
  - Membranes intact
  - Cephalic presentation, left occipito-transverse position
  - Station: 1 cm
  - Pelvis feels adequate

2 marks (½ mark for each point asked for)

Management
- Patient is in the active stage of labour
- Normal progress up until now

1 mark

- Continue with intermittent fetal auscultation
- (No need for IV access, urinary catheter, or continuous CTG monitoring – normal labour)
- Reassess with vaginal examination in 4 hours

1 mark

Q2
- First, examine the tocograph for the frequency of contractions (cannot tell the strength of contractions well from the CTG, but can assess their frequency)
- Baseline fetal heart rate (assessed between contractions): 100–160 bpm is reassuring
- Variability (variation in fetal heart rate around baseline): 5–10 bpm is reassuring
- Reactivity (accelerations in FHR over baseline): 2 accelerations of at least 15 bpm for at least 15 seconds each over a 20-minute period is reassuring
- Decelerations: absence of decelerations is reassuring

½ mark for each point (2½ marks total)

Q3
- Slow progress in the active phase of labour

1 mark

Assess the three 'Ps'
    Powers: contracting 2 in 10 mild
    Passenger: abdominal Ex (fetus does not feel large); vaginal Ex – no caput or moulding

Pelvis: vaginal Ex – pelvis feels adequate

3 marks (1 mark for each point)
- The slow progress is most likely due to poor contractions, based on the above assessment

1 mark
- Augment labour with an artificial rupture of membranes (ARM) +/– IV Syntocinon, and reassess vaginally in 4 hours. If no or little progress at that stage, may consider a caesarean section

2 marks
- Reassess need for pain relief. If inadequate, options include IM pethidine or an epidural

½ mark
20 marks total

Discussion

In this scenario the medical student is expected to demonstrate the ability to assess a normal labour, and then to manage slow progress in the active phase of labour.

The first stage of labour is from the onset of labour until full dilatation of the cervix. The second stage of labour is from full dilatation of the cervix until the delivery of the baby, and the third stage is from delivery of the baby until delivery of the placenta.

The first stage of labour is divided into the latent phase (from start of labour until cervix reaches dilatation of 4 cm) and active phase (from 4 cm until fully dilated). In the active phase of labour the normal rate of progress is roughly 1cm/hour in a primigravida.

The first scenario is of a woman at the start of a normal active phase of labour. In the third scenario, however, the labour is showing slow progress. Slow progress in the active phase of the first stage of labour requires an assessment of the three Ps: Powers (adequacy of uterine contractions), Passenger (size of fetus, signs of obstructed labour), and Pelvis (signs of a small/contracted pelvis on examination). If inadequate contractions, as in this case, augmentation of labour is indicated in the absence of other contraindications (e.g. fetal distress). If the 'passenger' is too large, or the 'pelvis' is too small, then delivery by caesarean section is indicated.

D4 Q1

The student is expected to take an adequate history and advise regarding how to use the combined oral contraceptive pill (COCP), and its benefits and risks.

History
- 24 years old
- Never pregnant
- Currently sexually active with one partner. Same partner for the last 3 months. Never been sexually active before. Using condoms but wants a method of contraception that is more certain

- Periods generally occur every 28 days, lasting 5 days with no problems; LMP 2 weeks ago
- No past history – medical or surgical. No contraindication to using the COCP
- Family history – mother developed breast cancer at age 54 years
- No allergies, no medications, non-smoker, occasional alcohol
- Never had a Pap smear
- Works as a secretary

5 marks

Q2
- Begin with a period
- Can start active pill on day 1 of cycle, which ensures immediate contraceptive protection
- If start non-active pill then need 7 active pills before safe
- COCP at same time each day to get into habit of using the COCP
- Side effects when starting include nausea, headaches, breast tenderness and breakthrough bleeding, which disappear within the first 3 months of starting
- 7-day rule for missed pills also applies if patient has vomiting, diarrhoea or is on antibiotics
- Must continue to use condoms to protect against viral sexually transmitted illnesses (STIs)

8 marks

Q3
Benefits
- Effective contraception
- Periods lighter and less painful. Less likely to become anaemic
- Less ovarian functional cysts
- Decreased risk of ovarian cancer
- Decreased risk of endometrial cancer
- Decreased incidence of bacterial STIs
- Fewer fibroids and endometriosis

Risks
- Deep venous thrombosis
- Increased gall bladder disease
- Probably no increase in breast cancer
- Small increase in cancer of the cervix

7 marks
20 marks total

Discussion
The COCP has two components – oestrogen (E) and progestagen (P). Ethinyl Oestradiol (EE) is a potent form of E and is present in every COCP. There are four different Ps used in the COCP. These are norethisterone

(NET) (first generation), laevonorgestrel (LNG) (second generation), norgestimate, desogestrel, and gestodene (all third generation) and cyproterone acetate (CPA) and drospirenone (both fourth generation).

The types of preparation include **monophasics**, **biphasics** and **triphasics**, depending on whether the dose of E and/or P remains constant throughout the cycle.

COCPs are further classified as high dose ($\geq$50 μg EE), low dose (<50 μg EE) or ultra low dose (20 μg EE).

The COCP is administered for 3 out of 4 weeks. It prevents ovulation by inhibiting gonadotrophin secretion via an effect on the hypothalamus and the pituitary. The P component suppresses LH and prevents ovulation and the E component suppresses FSH and prevents selection of a dominant follicle. The E provides stability to the endometrium and potentiates the action of the P component. The P component causes an atrophic endometrium, thick cervical mucus and decreases tubal motility. There is no evidence for a delay to return of fertility when the COCP is ceased.

With motivated subjects the annual failure rate with the COCP is 0.1%. Pregnancies usually occur when the week of placebo pills is prolonged with escape from ovarian suppression.

There are complications associated with the COCP. These include **venous thrombosis**. This is a dose-related effect of E with the highest incidence in the first year of use and the risk being limited to current users only, with a disappearance of risk 6 weeks after cessation. Varicose veins do not influence the risk of VTE development. The absolute risk of VTE is 1/10,000 women-years and is increased to 3–4/10,000 in a woman on the OCP. The relative risk of fatal pulmonary embolism in current users of the OCP is 9.6 with the absolute risk being 10.5/million women-years. It must be remembered that the risk of VTE in a pregnant woman is 30 times greater than in a non-pregnant woman.

The risk of **myocardial infarction** is increased in women over 35 years who *also* smoke. In these women the risk of death from the COCP is greater than the risk of death from pregnancy. The COCP acts synergistically with other risk factors for cardiovascular disease. For women over 35 years who do not smoke the benefits of the COCP far outweigh the risks. Women under 35 years, regardless of smoking status, are at no or only slightly increased risk of myocardial infaction. The risk of myocardial infarction is thought to be related to thromboembolic events rather than to an atherosclerotic event.

The overall risk of **stroke** in women of reproductive age is 5.5/100,000. There is an EE dose-dependent risk for the development of cerebral thromboembolic events, however, the low dose EE COCPs (<50 μg) do not increase this risk.

An increased incidence of clinically significant **hypertension** on the low dose pills has not been reported. If a woman has hypertension and it is well controlled on medication, the low dose COCP is not contraindicated.

Carbohydrate metabolism is affected mainly by the P component, but may also be partly affected by the EE influence on lipid metabolism, hepatic enzymes and the elevation of unbound cortisol. On the low dose formulations the changes are so mild as to be of no clinical significance. The COCP does not cause an increase in the incidence of diabetes.

Other metabolic effects include nausea, breast discomfort and bloating, as well as a possible decrease in libido, all of which are less evident with the low dose pills. Chloasma occurs in 5% and is becoming rarer with the lower doses of EE. But once it occurs it may never completely disappear.

The use of the COCP is protective for **endometrial cancer**. Use for at least 12 months reduces the risk by 50% with the greatest protection after 3 years of use and protection persists for 15 years after cessation. The risk of **ovarian cancer** is reduced by 40% and increases with the duration of use of the COCP (80% after 10 years) and continues for at least 10–15 years after discontinuation. There is a significant trend for the development of invasive **cervical cancer** with increasing duration of use of the COCP (RR 1.77 after 12 years of use). The risk appears to decline with increasing time after COCP discontinuation. The increased risk may occur because the COCP gives no protection against the human papilloma virus (HPV), but it has also been reported that in women with HPV there was a fourfold increase in the risk of cervical cancer compared with women not on the COCP who had HPV. Women on the COCP, like all women, should have regular cervical screening and should consider the HPV vaccine. Women who are currently using the COCP or have used it in the past 10 years are at a slightly increased risk of breast cancer diagnosis (RR 1.24 [1.15–1.33] current users; 1.07 [1.12–1.13] after 10 years). After 10 years of cessation of use there is no increase in the risk. More recently, no difference in breast cancer risk has been reported among current or past users of the COCP, no matter what age they began taking it, the dose of EE or the duration of use.

The risk of **bacterial STIs** is reduced by 50–60% in current users, but at least 12 months of use is necessary. This may be due to the alteration in the cervical mucus as well as to the reduction in menstrual blood loss. There is no protection against viral infections.

The **absolute contraindications** to the COCP include suspected pregnancy, thromboembolic disorders, cerebrovascular or coronary artery disease, markedly impaired liver function, a history of cholestatic jaundice, suspected breast cancer or other E-dependent neoplasia, herpes gestationis, a history of otosclerosis with known deterioration during pregnancy, undiagnosed abnormal vaginal bleeding, smokers over 35 years. A contraindication to the OCP is usually a contraindication to pregnancy.

Relative contraindications include migraines, uncontrolled hypertension, epilepsy (depending on the drugs used), sickle cell disease and active gall bladder disease. Provided there are no contraindications, a woman may use a low dose COCP until she reaches menopause.

If active pills are started on day 1 of the cycle there is immediate protection. If not started immediately then an additional form of contraception needs to be used for 7 active pill days. If a pill is missed (<12 h late) it should be taken as soon as remembered and the next taken as usual with no back-up required. If 2 are missed or greater than 12 h have elapsed, the forgotten pills should be taken and another form of contraception used for the next 7 active pill days. The most significant pills to miss are those that increase the length of the pill-free period. If this has occurred, the woman must miss the pill-free days and start a new pack immediately. If a woman has vomiting or diarrhoea or is taking antibiotics the COCP may not be absorbed adequately. She should be counselled on the 7-day rule.

For women who develop **breakthrough bleeding** or premenstrual symptoms on the COCP, reducing the pill-free interval to 3 days will often alleviate these symptoms. There is no reason that the COCP cannot be used **continuously** such that no withdrawal bleed occurs. The only problem may be breakthrough bleeding which usually disappears after one year of continuous use. This type of regimen is ideal in women with menstrual migraine or dysmennorrhoea.

Drugs may **decrease the plasma concentration of the COCP** by:
- inducing hepatic microsomal enzymes (rifampicin, some anticonvulsants)
- interfering with the enterohepatic recirculation of E (broad spectrum antibiotics), or interfering with absorption (antacids and purgatives).

Drugs that **increase COCP concentration** include high dose vitamin C. This is only of clinical significance if the vitamin C is stopped suddenly as there may be a rapid drop in COCP concentrations.

D5 Q1
History
- 40-year-old woman
- Planned, spontaneous pregnancy
- Was on folate, and rubella immunity has been checked (immune)
- 2 previous normal vaginal deliveries of term healthy babies (2 children, 7 years old and 5 years old)
- Blood group B negative, other antenatal screening tests by GP normal
- No gynae, medical or surgical history of note
- No family history of genetic problems
- Meds: folate; NKA
- Lives with husband; non-smoker, non-drinker; housewife

5 marks total, depending on completeness of history
(If asks for examination, direct to counsel regarding Down's risk: "What is my risk of Down syndrome, and how can we check for it?")

Counselling

Down syndrome is the most common chromosomal abnormality, resulting in intellectual disability, characterised by trisomy 21 (3 copies of chromosome 21).

Increasing maternal age is a major risk factor (roughly 1 in 1,500 at 20 y.o.; 1 in 300 at 36 y.o.; 1 in 100 at 40 y.o.; 1 in 40 at 44 y.o.).

Ninety-five per cent are sporadic mutations (non-dysjunction of maternal chromosomes during meiosis), but up to 5% are due to unbalanced translocations or mosaicism.

1½ marks

Q2

• An ultrasound has a low sensitivity for picking up Down syndrome.

1 mark

This patient should be offered non-invasive screening tests to determine the individual risk to her pregnancy of having Down syndrome. The options include:

1 nuchal translucency on ultrasound (11–13 weeks) – 70% sensitivity

2 marks

2 combined first trimester screening (nuchal translucency plus blood test for biochemical screening of βHCG and PAPP-A) – 80% sensitivity, 5% false positive

1½ marks

3 second trimester maternal serum screening (quadruple test) alphafetoprotein (↓ in T21), unconjugated estriol (↓ in T21), βHCG (↑ in T21), and Inhibin A (↑ in T21)
85% sensitivity (80% sensitivity if triple test without Inhibin A), 5% false positives

2 marks

Screening tests give an individual risk by adjusting age-related risk. They do not rule out Down syndrome completely, but allow patients to decide on whether they need an invasive diagnostic test or not.

2 marks

Q3

"You have a high-risk screening test for Down syndrome (anything more than 1 in 300 is considered high risk). This does not mean that the baby has Down syndrome. It does mean that invasive diagnostic tests are required to determine the exact chromosomes/karyotype of the baby." (or similar explanation)

1 mark

Options include:

1 chorionic villous sampling (CVS)
Can be performed 11–14 weeks (allows termination of pregnancy at earlier gestation), but 1% risk of miscarriage

1½ marks

2 amniocentesis
   15–18 weeks, 0.5% risk of miscarriage

1½ marks

N.B. For invasive tests this patient needs Anti-D immunoglobulin cover

1 mark

20 marks total

Discussion

In the past, Down syndrome testing with amniocentesis was only offered to women of advanced maternal age. However, most Down syndrome babies are born to women under 35 years old, as they are the women having the majority of the babies. The advent of non-invasive screening tests has revolutionised antenatal testing for Down syndrome. In the past, when only invasive diagnostic tests were available, their relatively high miscarriage risk limited their use to women at increased risk of Down syndrome pregnancies (i.e. maternal age and ultrasound markers). With the increasing age of women attempting to achieve a pregnancy at present, Down syndrome screening is a major obstetric issue for our patients.

A Down syndrome child has characteristic features:
• Slanted palpebral fissures; flat face; protruding tongue (macroglossia); hypotonia; loose skin on back of neck; single palmar crease; small general size

Down syndrome results in the following problems:
• Intellectual disability (mild to severe mental retardation, with no way of predicting the severity of retardation antenatally)
• Behavioural disturbances (especially at onset of puberty)
• Congenital malformations:
  – Heart malformations (30–40%) – ASD, VSD
  – Conductive deafness (60–80%)
  – Visual impairments: cataracts
  – Duodenal atresia
• Problems in later life:
  – Hypothyroidism: auto-immune thyroiditis
  – Susceptibility to infection
  – Leukemia (20-fold risk)
  – Early-onset Alzheimer's.

All women should be offered antenatal screening tests early in pregnancy, regardless of age. The woman must have a careful explanation as to what the test is for. The test should not be given to a woman who would carry on with the pregnancy regardless of the result (i.e. with moral or ethical objections to termination of pregnancy) as it will only cause anxiety, with no benefit to her or her baby.

In the OSCE case given, it would be acceptable to discuss the option of skipping the screening test altogether and going straight to a CVS or amniocentesis, given her age-related risk. However, she must be offered the

choice of a non-invasive screening test first, in case she wants to avoid the miscarriage risk associated with invasive needle tests.

While the better students will be able to name the hormones tested in the serum screening tests, as well as sensitivity and false positive rates, it is not necessary in order to obtain the marks allocated in this OSCE.

D6 Q1

History
- 20-year-old nulliparous woman
- Regular menstrual cycle on combined oral contraceptive pill
- LMP 1/52 ago
- Single episode of post-coital bleeding: bright loss immediately after intercourse; some lower abdominal discomfort associated with the bleeding
- No previous episodes of PCB; no intermenstrual bleeding (IMB)
- No dysuria, dyspareunia
- Some occasional vaginal discharge (non-offensive) in last couple of weeks
- Sexually active since age 17 (3 partners, current boyfriend of 1 month)
- No history of genital warts/herpes
- Never had a Pap smear
- No significant past medical/surgical history
- NKA; medications (COCP)
- University student (arts/law); smokes 10 cigarettes per day; alcohol on weekends; no recreational drugs

7 marks, depending on completeness of history

Q2
- Pap smear
- Post-coital bleeding, therefore needs a colposcopic examination as well as a Pap smear
- High vaginal swab for M/C/S
- Endocervical swab for chlamydia/gonorrhoea
- First catch urine for chlamydia/gonorrhoea PCR (test for DNA of the organisms)

3 marks total (1 mark for 1 of above, 2 marks for 3 of above, 2½ marks for 4 of above, 3 marks for all 5)

Q3
- Chlamydia treatment options:
  – Azithromycin 1g PO stat
  OR
  – Doxycycline 100mg BD PO 7–10 days

2 marks

- Counsel regarding side effects of treatment (gastrointestinal symptoms, doxycycline best taken with food)

½ mark

- Notifiable disease: must complete relevant paperwork to DHS

½ mark

- Partner must be treated regardless of absence of symptoms to prevent reinfection
- Options for telling partner:
  – Patient may advise partner herself
  – Doctor may tell partner directly with patient's consent
  – Partner may be contacted by DHS partner notifying officer with consent of the patient (patient identity not disclosed)

2 marks

Education

- Patient should be given information on sexually transmitted infections (STIs) and their transmission
- Encourage reduced risk by using condoms
- Advise to refrain from sexual intercourse for 7 days after single dose therapy, or until completion of a 7-day regimen **and** until all their sexual partners have been treated
- Should be advised of heath risks from smoking, and encouraged to quit

2½ marks

Follow-up:

- Re-evaluate for signs and symptoms
- Treat reinfection if it occurs
- Reinforce safe sex practice
- Recommend serology for HIV, hepatitis B, and syphilis (now, and in 3/12 time)
- Test of cure is only needed if pregnant (dependent on compliance)
- Re-screen in 3–4 months

2½ marks
20 marks total

Discussion

The student is expected to take a relevant sexual history, perform the appropriate investigations, and counsel the patient as outlined in the ideal answer. The patient presents with vaginal discharge and an episode of post-coital bleeding. Post-coital bleeding mandates a colposcopic examination of the cervix, not just a Pap smear (which is a screening test only, not a diagnostic test). The history of unprotected sexual intercourse with a new boyfriend, as well as recent onset of vaginal discharge, should prompt the student to screen for STDs.

The treatment of a chlamydial infection is outlined in the ideal answer above.

D7 Q1

Antenatal testing required and rationale

Blood group and antibodies

- If Rhesus negative, need repeated testing for development of antibodies against Rhesus +ve babies, which can harm pregnancy, and anti-D immunoglobulin administration antenatally and postnatally to prevent isoimmunisation, which could harm future pregnancies
- Presence of other antibodies needs increased monitoring in case it could affect the pregnancy

Full blood examination

- Pregnant women at risk of iron deficiency anaemia (would need iron supplementation). Other haemoglobinopathies need to be detected as may have implications for maternal and fetal health

Syphilis testing (e.g. Rapid Plasma Reagin test)

- If positive, need treatment with penicillin to prevent congenital syphilis in the fetus

Hepatitis B serology

- If hep B +ve, need active and passive immunisation of the newborn (hep B vaccination and immunoglobulins) to prevent hepatitis B of the newborn

Rubella serology

- If the mother contracts rubella (German measles) during pregnancy, can have severe congenital defects of the baby. Low immune or non-immune women need to have a vaccination post-partum (cannot give vaccine when pregnant)

HIV serology

- Should be offered antenatally to **all** women. If HIV +ve, steps can be taken to reduce risk of vertical transmission from 30% to 2% (zidovudine or AZT to mother antenatally and to infant post-partum, elective caesarean section rather than vaginal delivery, and no breastfeeding)

MSU

- Pregnant women at increased risk of urinary tract infections, and often asymptomatic. Early detection and treatment reduces risk of miscarriage and PPROM, as well as pyelonephritis in the mother

Vitamin D/calcium

- Fully veiled women, particularly from Muslim migrant backgrounds, can be at risk of vitamin D deficiency due to lack of sun exposure. Needs to have vitamin D supplementation if deficient

Down syndrome screening

- Should be offered to **all** pregnant women after discussion about what they would do if they had a positive screen (Mrs Hassim does not want it)

9 marks (½ mark for listing each test, further ½ for each correct explanation)

2 marks general competency for counselling in lay terms

Q2

The exam candidate should recognise that the results are all normal, apart from the low mean cell volume (MCV) on the full blood examination, and the low vitamin D levels.

2 marks

It should be explained to the patient that the low MCV could mean either:
- iron deficiency – need iron studies to confirm; If low iron, need iron supplementation and rechecked FBE at least once per trimester

2 marks

or

- haemoglobinopathy (e.g. thalassaemia) – need to be checked with haemoglobin electrophoresis (for beta thalassaemia) and possibly DNA testing with PCR (alpha thalassaemia).

2 marks

- Need partner testing with FBE – if normal, no risk of major haemoglobinopathies in the fetus; if abnormal, need to refer for genetic counselling regarding risks of the fetus inheriting a major haemoglobinopathy

1 mark

- The low vitamin D levels mean that Mrs Hassim needs vitamin D replacement (Ostelin tablets 2 per day), and needs to have her vitamin D levels rechecked in 3 months.

2 marks

20 marks total

Discussion

This station tests the ability of the student not only to know what routine antenatal tests are performed at the first antenatal visit, but why they are performed, as well as the ability to explain this to the patient in lay terms she can understand. This is an important skill in clinical practice. In general, if a patient understands why she is being tested and the benefit to her pregnancy, she is more likely to comply with testing. The doctor must have a basic understanding of the implications of abnormal results, and how they change the management of a normal pregnancy.

The second part of the OSCE tests the student's knowledge of causes for a low mean cell volume of red blood cells on full blood examination. The possibility of a haemoglobinopathy, as well as the more common iron deficiency anaemia, needs to be considered, especially in view of the higher risk of this due to the presented patient's migrant background.

It has been shown that women from cultural backgrounds which advocate extensively covering their bodies, such as those from veiled Muslim cultures, especially dark-skinned women, are at risk of vitamin D deficiency. In a study of these women attending a Melbourne antenatal clinic it was shown that 80% had a vitamin D level below the test reference range, putting them at risk of bone disease and of neonatal hypoglycaemia in their children (Grover & Mori 2001). This needs to be considered in the patient in this OSCE, as well as the routine tests listed.

Long-term vitamin D deficiency is associated with heart disease and breast cancer, as well as increased risk of intrauterine growth restriction and premature labour in pregnant women. If a child is born into a vitamin D deficient household, there is the later risk of rickets and osteomalacia.

Reference
Grover S, Morely R 2001 Vitamin D deficiency in veiled or dark-skinned pregnant women. Medical Journal of Australia 175:251–252

D8 Q1
History
- 46-year-old woman
- Bleeding every 2 weeks for the past 6 months, lasting 4–5 days
- Periods regular prior to this
- Soaks through tampons and heavy pads, needing to change pads every 2 hours on days 1–2
- Dysmenorrhoea, especially in the first 2 days
- Tired, decreased exercise tolerance
- G4P3 – three normal vaginal deliveries (children aged 5, 8 and 10), one 8/40 miscarriage
- Laparoscopic tubal ligation aged 40 y.o.
- Last Pap smear 4 years ago (normal; no abnormal smears in past)

Medical problems
- Hypertension (Rx with ACE inhibitor)
- Hypercholesterolaemia (Rx lipitor)

Past surgery
- Laparoscopic cholecystectomy
- Appendicectomy (18 years old)
- Family Hx: mother alive and well (83 years old); Father died of prostate cancer 72 y.o.
- Allergic to penicillin (anaphylactic reaction as a child); Meds as above
- Housewife/mother; non-smoker; drinks a glass of wine/night

6 marks, depending on completeness of history

Q2
Examination
- Signs of anaemia – conjunctiva, palmar creases (both pale)
- BP 120/70, pulse rate 92 bpm
- BMI 27
- Thyroid/breast Ex: normal
- Cardiac Ex: dual heart sounds, nil added
- Abdominal Ex: normal
- Vulva: normal in appearance
- Speculum Ex: cervix normal, Pap smear taken; can take Pipelle sample of endometrium

- Bimanual pelvic Ex: bulky, anteverted uterus, no adnexal masses
  5 marks depending on completeness (1 mark for suggesting a pipelle sample of endometrium)

Q3
- Full blood examination
- Iron studies
- Urea, electrolytes and creatinine
- Liver function tests
- Thyroid function tests
- Pelvic ultrasound scan
  3 marks (½ mark for each investigation)

Q4
- If no pipelle sample taken, next step given the thickened endometrial lining and the history is a hysteroscopy, D+C
  1 mark

Management
- Medroxyprogesterone acetate: 10 mg/day for 14 days per month
  OR
- Mirena IUD insertion

Side effects of medroxyprogesterone acetate:
- Headaches
- Breast tenderness/pain
- Mood swings/irritability
- Abdominal bloating
- Irregular/breakthrough bleeding

Side effects of Mirena:
- Irregular bleeding for first few months
  5 marks
  20 marks total

Discussion
The student is expected to be able to adequately assess the presenting problem, order the appropriate investigations and discuss treatment options. The patient presented has endometrial hyperplasia. Her risk factors include her age and the fact that she is overweight (BMI = 27). Her adipose tissue acts as an extra source of estrogen, increasing her risk of endometrial hyperplasia and cancer. The endometrial lining is abnormally thickened on ultrasound investigation at 20 mm, which should prompt the student to perform an endometrial sampling, either by pipelle or by a curettage at the time of a hysteroscopy. The lack of atypical cells of the histopathology of her endometrium makes conservative medical treatment the best option.

5

Specialist level practice OSCE questions

MRANZCOG OSCE E

E1 Q1

Letter

Dear Doctor,

I am referring Mrs Harvey, a 26-year-old woman with a kidney transplant, to you for advice, as she wishes to start her family. Please advise and manage her.

Regards

Dr N Ephron

Q2

Mrs Harvey returns for the results of her tests.

Investigation results

- U+E+Cr normal, apart from mildly elevated creatinine (130 μmol/L)
- MSU neg
- 24-hour urine creatinine – normal
- 24-hour urine protein – 0.12 g
- Rubella immune
- Pap smear normal
- Antihypertensive changed to Aldomet (methyldopa) by renal physician

"Can I start trying for a pregnancy, doctor?"

Q3

How will your management of her pregnancy differ from a normal pregnancy?

Q4

Mrs Harvey is 23^{+3} weeks pregnant, and was admitted to the ward with pre-eclampsia 2 weeks ago. You are the resident on night duty and have been called by the midwives to see her as she is feeling unwell with abdominal pain. Please manage.

E2 Encounter 1

Mrs M presents with a 3-month history of post-menopausal bleeding.

Please take an appropriate history from Mrs M.

Encounter 2

Please ask for relevant examination findings. What investigations would you order?

Encounter 3

The patient presents a week later for the results of her investigations.

Investigation results

- FBE: Haemoglobin 110 g/dl, normal white cell count and platelets
- U+E+Cr: normal, creatinine 105
- LFTs: normal
- HbA1C: 10%
- Pelvic ultrasound: Anteverted uterus measuring 80 mm length × 45 mm A–P × 50 mm width. The cervix is normal in appearance. The uterus is mobile and non-tender. The endometrium is thickened, measuring 15 mm, with increased vascularity. The right ovary measures 17 × 16 × 19 mm, is mobile and non-tender. The left ovary could not be identified. No adnexal mass is seen. There is no pelvic free fluid. Conclusion: thickened endometrium.

"What do we do now, doctor?"

Encounter 4

You are now seeing Mrs M following her hysteroscopy/D+C.

- Histopathology of uterine curettings: Grade 2 endometrial adenocarcinoma

"Doctor, what are the results from my test? Do I have cancer? Am I going to die?"

E3 Encounter 1

You are the obstetric registrar on call for a tertiary level labour ward. A midwife calls you for a Mrs CK, who has been pushing for 2 hours in second stage, and now has an abnormal CTG. Please manage.

Encounter 2

With the third pull of the forceps the head of the baby is delivered, but the shoulders are stuck. How do you proceed?

Encounter 3

Following delivery of the baby, Mrs CK has had a post-partum haemorrhage, which is being managed with oxytocics, as well as IV resuscitation with whole blood. Half an hour later the bleeding has been controlled and the midwife calls you back to the labour ward: "Mrs CK is distressed with fever, chills, and chest discomfort with wheezing!" Please advise on your management.

Encounter 4

Mrs CK's baby was successfully delivered, with a birthweight of 3.7 kg, but her baby appears to have a brachial plexus palsy. You are now seeing her on the postnatal ward. Please counsel both with regards to her baby and any implications for her next pregnancy.

E4 Encounter 1
Letter

Mr and Mrs F are unable to become pregnant after trying for 5 years. Could you please advise them regarding their options.

Encounter 2

Mr and Mrs F return 6 weeks later to discuss the results of their tests.

Test results
- Days 2–4 FSH 4IU/L
  - LH 4IU/L
  - Oestradiol 80 pmol/L
- TSH 1.45
- Mid luteal progesterone 40 nmol/L
- Rubella immune, varicella immune
- SA+IBT: 45 million/mL, 50% forward motility, 80% abnormal forms, negative IBT

"Is there anything else to be done, doctor?"

Encounter 3

A diagnostic laparoscopy is performed and the patient is discovered to have severe endometriosis with a 4 cm left endometrioma. The anatomy is distorted with both ovaries adherent in the POD with bowel overlying, the fimbrial ends of both tubes are not present within the adhesions. The tubes are patent, the hysteroscopy is normal.

"What do you advise, doctor?"

Encounter 4

The operation proceeded well, and you advised the couple to try for a pregnancy for 6 months before coming to see you again.

The couple re-present as pregnancy has not occurred after 6 months of regular sexual intercourse.

"Is there anything we can do to start our family, doctor?"

E5 Encounter 1

You have been asked to do the elective caesarean section list at a tertiary hospital for a colleague who is ill. The first case is a 32-year-old woman, Mrs M, gravida 4 para 3, with a suspected placenta percreta.

The patient, Mrs M, is in the theatre reception area. Please take a brief history from her.

Encounter 2
For which investigations would you like to see the results? What should have been done prior to delivery?

Encounter 3
Investigation results
- Haemoglobin 98 g/dl
- U+E+creatinine, coagulation profile normal
- Urinalysis: no blood
- Ultrasound: shows anterior placenta invading the full thickness of the myometrium with a suggestion of invasion into the bladder
- MRI: shows possible bladder invasion

What are the alternative options for management of the placenta in this case?

Encounter 4
You proceed to surgery. To attempt to decrease blood loss you decide to ligate the internal iliac arteries. Describe how you would go about this.

Encounter 5
What are the branches of the internal iliac artery, and what are the potential complications of dividing the posterior branch?

E6 ### Encounter 1
Mrs B, a fit and sprightly 80-year-old woman, is referred to you by her GP after he has tried unsuccessfully to treat her vulval itch.

Please take an appropriate history from Mrs B.

Encounter 2
Please ask for relevant examination findings.

Encounter 3
What investigations would you like to perform?

Encounter 4
The vulval biopsy shows squamous cell carcinoma of the vulva (SCC). The other investigations are normal. There is no evidence of groin node enlargement on the CT scan.

What is the most appropriate management?

Encounter 5
You have referred Mrs B to a gynaecological oncologist, but she wants to know why, what will they do next, and are there any risks involved?

E7 ### Encounter 1
Letter
Thank you for seeing Miss B, a 25-year-old woman who presents with a 2-year history of irregular periods. Please manage her problem.

Encounter 2

The patient returns 4 weeks later for the test results. She still has not had a period.

Test results

- FSH 4 IU/L
- LH 16 IU/L
- Prolactin 400 mIU/mL (0–600 mIU/L)
- Testosterone 3.5 nmol/L (0.2–2.8 nmol/L)
- DHEAS 13 µmol/L (2–11µmol/L)
- TSH 2.5 (0.4–5.0)
- FAI 12 (<5)
- SHBG 10 (20–200)

Ultrasound

- The uterus is not enlarged. The endometrium has a non-specific appearance and measures 8 mm
- Each ovary contains between 40–50 follicles. There are no cysts in either of the ovaries.

"What do the results show, doctor?" Please discuss results and any further tests required.

"Are there any long-term health risks associated with my condition, doctor?"

Encounter 3

Further test results.

GTT: Fasting 4 mmol/L
   – 1 hour: 8 mmol/L
   – 2 hour: 6 mmol/L

- Cholesterol 6.6 mmol/L (<5.5 mmol/L)
- Triglyceride 1.5 mmol/L (<2.5 mmol/L)
- HDL 1.2 mmol/L (>2.5 mmol/L)
- LDL 3.8 mmol/L (<3.5 mmol/L)

Discuss the results of the further tests with Miss B.

"Is there anything that can be done to reduce the hair growth, doctor?"

"Are there any other treatments necessary for my condition?"

E8 Q1

You are seeing Mrs Bertram in antenatal clinic for her first antenatal visit, with a twin pregnancy from IVF (in-vitro fertilisation).

Please take a history and advise on management.

Q2

Mrs Bertram is returning to the clinic for the results of her Down syndrome screening test.

- Blood group: A neg, no antibodies
- FBE: Hb 130 MCV 86 platelets 197
- HepBsAg: neg
- Rubella: immune
- TPHA: negative
- HIV: negative
- MSU: no growth on culture
- Down syndrome screening by nuchal translucency for twins:
  - Normal nuchal translucency for twin 1
  - Increased nuchal translucency for twin 2
- First trimester maternal serum screen: increased T21 risk
- Combined screening risk result: 1 in 80

"What do we do now, doctor?"

Q3
The result from the amniocentesis shows trisomy 21 in the second twin, and 46XY normal in the first twin.

Please counsel Mrs Bertram regarding her options.

MRANZCOG OSCE F

F1 Encounter 1
A 28-year-old woman, Mrs K, is referred to you with a history of right iliac fossa pain for 6 months. A pelvic ultrasound scan has shown a 14 cm solid mass arising from the right ovary.

Please take an appropriate history from Mrs K.

Encounter 2
Please ask for relevant examination findings.

Encounter 3
What investigations would you like to order?

Encounter 4
Mrs K cancelled her follow-up visit to discuss her results, as she had an important meeting to attend interstate. On her return, she was driving back from the airport when she developed acute abdominal pain. Her husband drove her to the Emergency Department and you have been asked to attend.

What would be your management on arrival?

Encounter 5
At laparotomy, a ruptured haemorrhagic right ovarian mass was removed. The mass appeared to be predominantly blood clot. The left tube, ovary and the uterus looked normal. The abdomen was irrigated with warm saline thoroughly to remove the blood. All peritoneal surfaces were inspected, as

well as the bowel, liver, spleen and stomach. Lymph nodes were checked (none enlarged). The incision was closed.

Final histology: Granulosa cell tumour
Had the patient not had an emergency operation for an acute abdomen, and had you known that the initial blood results had shown a raised Inhibin B (2492 pg/mL), what would have been the appropriate surgical management for this woman, who wishes to preserve her fertility if possible?

Encounter 6
If the patient had atypical endometrial hyperplasia and Stage 1A germ-cell tumour, what would be your future management?

F2 Encounter 1
Letter
Thank you for seeing Miss A, a 16-year-old who presents with primary amenorrhoea. Please manage her problem.

Encounter 2
The patient returns 4 weeks later for the test results. She still has not had a period.

Test results
- FSH: 4 IU/L
- LH: 4 IU/L
- Estradiol 400 pmol/L
- Progesterone 50 nmol/L
- Prolactin 400 mIU/mL (0–600 mIU/L)

Ultrasound
A transabdominal scan was performed. The uterus is not present and there is no vaginal stripe. Both ovaries are seen and there are 10 follicles in each ovary.

She and her mother ask: "What is the diagnosis?"

"Is there any treatment necessary?"

"What are the options for future child-bearing?"

F3 Encounter 1
You are called down to the Emergency Department to see Ms Thorburn, a 24-year-old primigravida at 22 weeks gestation. The resident informs you of a 1-day history of severe central chest pain associated with shortness of breath. Please assess and manage.
The examiner will play the role of the patient.
What is your differential diagnosis? What investigations will you order?

Encounter 2

The emergency resident calls you back down to casualty 2 hours later. The results of your tests are available.

Test results

- Arterial blood gases: PH 7.40 pCO2 22 PO2 68
- CXR normal
- VQ high probability pulmonary embolus
- ECG Sinus tachycardia nil else
- Spiral CT saddle pulmonary embolus
- Blood for procoagulants: FVL, Pr C/PrS, ATIII, LAC, ACL, Prothrombin gene mutation (pending) – may be ordered after diagnosis of pulmonary embolus

Outline your management.

Encounter 3

The treatment of the pulmonary embolus is successful. Mrs Thorburn is still on Clexane treatment and is now seeing you for management in the antenatal clinic at 38 weeks gestation.

Encounter 4

You are in the recovery room of the operating theatre, having performed a LUSCS for obstructed labour 30 minutes ago. The recovery nurse approaches you saying that she is worried about the blood loss, which has been 100 mL since the return from theatre.

In the recovery room (you are in attendance) the examiner plays the role of the recovery nurse.

F4   Q1

You are the O&G specialist on duty, and you are called to see Miss Bennett, a 22-year-old sex worker, who has presented to the Emergency Department with a vulval ulceration.

Please assess and manage.

Q2

The results of your tests and investigations are as follows:

- B-HCG 39,000
- Pelvic ultrasound: singleton intrauterine pregnancy 15/40 gestation, placenta not low, liquor normal, ovaries normal
- TPHA +ve
- VDRL/RPR +ve titre 1:128
- HVS normal vaginal flora
- Culture/immunofluorescence from ulcer –ve
- Dark-field microscopy/silver staining from ulcer: spirochaetes seen
- HSV IgG +ve, HSV IgM –ve
- Cervical/urethral/anal swabs –ve for gonorrhoea/chlamydia
- Hepatitis B serology –ve

- Hepatitis C serology +ve
- HIV serology −ve
- Pap smear normal

Outline your management.

Q3

Miss Bennett is on a stable dose of methadone and has stopped using heroin. Her VDRL/RPR levels have dropped to titres of 1:8 with treatment.

She presents to the labour ward at term in early labour with ruptured membranes 3 hours ago. Last night she had an eruption of painful genital ulcers.

What is your management?

F5 Encounter 1

Letter: Mr and Mrs E are unable to become pregnant after trying for 3 years and they are very anxious about this. Could you please advise them regarding their options.

Encounter 2

Mr and Mrs E return 6 weeks later to discuss the results of your investigations.

Test results
- Days 2–4 FSH 4 IU/L
  - LH 4 IU/L
  - Oestradiol 80 pmol/L
- TSH 1.45
- Mid luteal progesterone 40 nmol/L
- Rubella immune
- Varicella immune
- SA+IBT azospermia

Encounter 3

Mr E returns to see you with his wife for the results of your further investigations.

Test results
- Male FSH 5 IU/l
- LH 4 IU/L
- Prolactin 400 mIU/mL
- Testosterone 20 nmol/L
- Karyotype 46 XY
- Cystic fibrosis carrier for Delta F 508 gene mutation
- Cystic fibrosis testing for female shows carrier Delta F 508 gene mutation.

"Is there anything we can do to have a baby, doctor?"

F6   Encounter 1

You receive a letter regarding a patient presenting to your rooms:

Dear doctor,
Could you please perform a Pap smear for Georgia Melton, a 22-year-old woman, who is due for her first Pap smear. I was unable to perform a Pap smear in the rooms, as she found it too painful. Thank you for your assistance.
Regards
Dr LMO

The patient has presented with her husband.

Encounter 2a

"What's wrong with me doctor? I know that this isn't normal. Can anything be done about it? What sort of operation will help me?"

Encounter 2b

"How are we going to have babies if we can't have sex?"

F7   Q1

You are seeing Mrs Brock for her first antenatal visit. You have the following letter:

Dear Dr,
Would you please take over the management of Mrs Brock, a 25-year-old woman who is 8 weeks by dates. She has a history of heart valve disease due to rheumatic fever in childhood.
Regards
Dr LMO

Q2

Mrs Brock goes into spontaneous labour at 37/40. She is transferred to the cardiac ward for cardiac monitoring with a midwife in attendance. Her labour has progressed well, and she has just started pushing. You are now called to the labour ward to see her by the midwife, as Mrs Brock has become acutely unwell with difficulty breathing associated with drowsiness. At the same time the CTG is now showing late decelerations.

Q3

Post-partum, Mrs Brock has a 2-week stay in the intensive care unit. She required a blood transfusion while in the ICU. After her discharge she was discovered to have developed anti-Kell antibodies.

Counsel her about the risk these pose, if any, to her subsequent pregnancies.

F8   Q1

You have been referred a 16-year-old girl, Miss T, who presents with her mother, by her local doctor, with the following letter:

Dear Doctor
Thank you for seeing Miss T a 16-year-old who presents with primary amenorrhoea. Please manage her problem.
Regards
Dr LMO

Q2

Miss T is now returning to see you 4 weeks later for her test results. She still has not had a period.

- FSH: 4 IU/L
- LH: 20 IU/L
- Prolactin: 400 mIU/mL (0–600 mIU/L)
- Testosterone: 10 nmol/L
- Estradiol: 400 pmol/L
- DHEAS: 10 nmol/L
- Progesterone: 2 nmol/L

Ultrasound

- A transabdominal scan was performed. The uterus is not present and there is no vaginal stripe. Neither ovaries are seen.
- Karyotype 46XY

"What do my test results show, doctor?"

MRANZCOG OSCE G

G1 Q1
You are the obstetrics registrar on duty in the evening at a tertiary hospital. Mrs White has been sent in to the casualty by a nearby imaging centre with an ultrasound reporting the following:

- A 18/40 intrauterine singleton pregnancy with signs of moderate fetal hydrops. Placenta is clear of the os. Normal ovaries.

Please assess the patient and outline your management.

Q2

You are a consultant in the materno-fetal medicine unit, and are seeing Mrs White with the results of her investigations. They are as follows:

- Hb electrophoresis: no abnormal peaks, normal
- HbA1C: 4.7
- Liver function tests: normal
- Kleihauer test: negative
- Blood group and antibodies: O neg, no antibodies
- Parvovirus IgM +ve IgG +ve
- Rubella IgM –ve IgG –ve
- CMV IgM –ve IgG –ve
- HepBsAg –ve
- Toxoplasma IgM –ve IgG –ve

- Repeat tertiary unit ultrasound: no fetal anomalies seen, fetal hydrops again noted
- Amniocentesis: 46XX on FISH analysis, karyotype still pending, no growth on culture

You are counselling the patient regarding the results.

Q3

Unfortunately, Mrs White's fetus is found to have no fetal cardiac activity at the time of the intra-uterine transfusion. She has elected to have a dilatation and evacuation of the dead fetus, which you are performing.

At surgery, a major perforation of the uterine fundus is suspected. What is your management?

Q4

A large fundal perforation is found at laparoscopy, but no damage to bowel or other intraperitoneal organs. She requires a laparotomy to suture the fundus.

You are seeing Mrs White post-operatively.

G2 Encounter 1

You are the gynaecologist on call for a country hospital and you are called by the Emergency Department regarding Miss M, a 15-year-old girl, who has presented to the department with pain and an obvious abdominal mass.

What aspects of the history and examination would you like to ask over the phone to the emergency doctor ?

Encounter 2

For which investigations would you like the results?

Encounter 3
Investigation results

- FBE Hb 90 g/dl, WCC 14.0
- U+E+Cr, LFT, coagulation profile: all normal
- CXR: bilateral atelectasis
- CT scan: cystic mass arising from pelvis separate from uterus, likely ovarian in origin; some septations seen
- Beta-HCG negative; LDH normal
- Other tumour markers not yet available

You have attended the emergency and have reviewed Miss M. She is there with her mother. Both are anxious. What is your management?

Encounter 4

The final histopathology has shown a low-grade borderline serous tumour of the right ovary. A successful ovarian cystectomy was performed, with the cyst removed intact.

What do you recommend next and why?

Encounter 5

Miss M returns for a routine follow-up. She has declined to take the oral contraceptive pill and has been having 6-monthly ultrasound scans for 2 years, but then does not attend for 18 months. Her GP has arranged a pelvic ultrasound scan, which has shown a 5 cm cyst on the right ovary. What is your management?

G3 ### Encounter 1
Letter

Thank you for seeing Miss M, a 6-year-old who presents with Turner's syndrome. She will be starting on growth hormone shortly. Her mother is interested in the way in which secondary sexual characteristics will be developed and wants to know what long-term investigations will need to be performed. She also wants to know about her daughter's options for future fertility.

The examiner will play the role of the patient's mother. No further history needs to be taken.

The mother asks, "My daughter will be treated with growth hormone to increase her height. How will breast development occur?"

Encounter 2

The mother asks, "What are the health implications for my daughter, and what tests need to be done in the future?"

Encounter 3

The mother asks, "What are the options for fertility for my daughter? If she gets pregnant are there any risks to the pregnancy?"

Encounter 4

(Direct question from examiner to candidate)

"Doctor, I have been reading about Turner's syndrome on the internet, and am curious about how the clinical presentation and/or your management would differ if my daughter was:
- a 45X/46XX mosaic?
- a 45X/46XY mosaic?"

G4 ### Encounter 1

You are the on-call obstetrician at a large, isolated provincial hospital, and have just been rung by a general practitioner. A woman at 26 weeks gestation with a blood pressure of 190/110 has been referred to the midwifery unit for admission. The prior blood pressures have always been <140/90, and the blood pressure at the first visit was 110/60.

You are in the unit and meet the patient, Mrs Cook. Take a history and outline your management.

Encounter 2

You have arranged to transfer Mrs Cook to a level 3 hospital by air ambulance, but the weather has closed the airport and it is unlikely to open until the following day. You get a phone call at 2300 hrs from the midwifery ward to say that the fetal heart is only 80 bpm.

Outline your management.

Encounter 3

The patient has been transferred to ICU, intubated and started on a nitroprusside infusion. The fetus dies and the ICU staff are having trouble controlling her blood pressure and weaning her off the ventilator.

Outline your plan of management.

Encounter 4

On vaginal examination the cervix is long, hard and closed. Prostaglandin pessaries are used over a 4-day period, with no change in the cervix and no uterine activity. The patient's blood pressure is still difficult to control, and she is still being ventilated.

Outline your management.

Encounter 5

You perform a LUSCS and deliver a still-born baby. The post-operative course is uneventful. On the 6th day post-op she is ready to be discharged when you are called to her room and find her lying on the floor of her room, cyanosed, with a BP of 60/20.

Outline your management.

G5 Encounter 1

Mrs D presents with hot flushes and night sweats and wants to discuss HT with you. She has not had a period for 12 months. Please manage her problem.

Encounter 2

Mrs D returns to see you 6 weeks later. "What do my test results show, doctor? Do I need to do anything about them?"

Test results
- Bone density: T score spine −1.75, T score hip −1.5
- Vitamin D 30 (75–250)

Encounter 3

"Is there any treatment for my hot flushes?"

G6 Encounter 1

Mrs KL presents to your clinic with the following letter:

Dear Dr,
Mrs KL is a 32-year-old woman with regular painful menstrual bleeding. Could you please manage her problem?
Yours sincerely
Dr GP

Encounter 2
The decision is made to proceed with a diagnostic laparoscopy and hysteroscopy. Please describe your technique for commencing the surgery.

Encounter 3
At surgery, a normal uterine cavity and lining are found at hysteroscopy, with normal endometrium on histopathology. At laparoscopy, endometriosis is diagnosed, with bilateral pelvic side wall endometriosis as well as a large rectovaginal nodule, obliterating the Pouch of Douglas.

You are seeing Mrs KL 2 weeks later. Advise her on management.

Encounter 4
You are operating with your registrar, who asks you, "What are the types of electrosurgical injuries possible during laproscopic surgery?"

Encounter 5
Laproscopic surgery to excise the rectovaginal nodule is successful, with no complications. Mrs KL recovers well and is discharged from hospital the next day.

It is now 6 months later, and you are seeing Mrs KL in your rooms for a follow-up appointment. She is complaining of left-sided pelvic pain. Please advise on your management.

G7 Encounter 1
Ms P, a 26-year-old woman, presents to the Emergency Department with vaginal bleeding at 14 weeks gestation.

Please take an appropriate history from Ms P.

Encounter 2
You have examined the patient. She has a mild systolic murmur, is tachycardic, but her blood pressure is within normal limits. Her mucous membranes are dry and her uterus is 16 weeks size. No fetal heart is heard with doppler. What investigations would you like to order?

Encounter 3
- FBE and U+E+creatinine suggest the patient is dehydrated. The ultrasound scan is reported as showing areas of relative hypoechogenicity and hyperechogenicity. No fetus or gestational sac are seen.
- Beta-HCG is 500,000 IU/L

What do you tell the patient, and what is your management?

Encounter 4

The histopathology from your suction curettage shows a complete hydatidiform molar pregnancy.

Please explain the features of a complete versus a partial mole, including the genetic features.

Encounter 5

What is your management following curettage?

Encounter 6

The beta-HCG levels are as follows:

- Week 1 post curettage: 10,000 IU/L
- Week 2: 5,000 IU/L
- Week 3: 1,000 IU/L
- Week 4: 4,250 IU/L

What is your management?

Encounter 7

There is no evidence of metastatic disease. What is your management?

G8 Q1

You are doing a private obstetric locum in a small private hospital and are called by the midwives to see Mrs Beresford, a 31-year-old woman with twins conceived after IVF treatment. She has been complaining of slight, fresh PV bleeding since this morning.

Please assess and manage.

Q2

The ambulance arrives to take Mrs Beresford to the nearest tertiary obstetric hospital, with you as escort. While in transit, in the back of the ambulance, the membranes rupture and a loop of cord appears at the introitus.

What is your management?

Q3

You arrive at the tertiary hospital 15 minutes later and rush to theatre. Describe how you would perform the classical caesarean section.

Q4

It is now 12 weeks since the dramatic delivery of the twins, and Mrs Beresford is seeing you in your rooms with her husband. He tells you that she has been tearful and moody of late, and is having trouble managing the twins.

Please assess and manage.

MRANZCOG OSCE H

H1 Encounter 1

Mrs Brown presents to your surgery with the following letter:

Dear Dr,

Please take care of Mrs Brown, a 50-year-old woman with worsening urinary incontinence. I would like you to take over the management of this problem.

Regards

Dr LMO

Encounter 2

The results of your tests come back as follows:

- Mid-stream urine culture – negative
- Urodynamics – severe urodynamic stress incontinence with a mild degree of detrusor overactivity/urge incontinence

"What can we do to fix the problem, doctor?"

Encounter 3

It is now 6 weeks after your operation. Mrs Brown has come to your rooms for a follow-up visit, complaining of vaginal discharge.

Encounter 4

At a follow-up visit 1 year later Mrs Brown presents complaining of an itchy, sore vulva. Please assess and manage.

H2 Q1

You are the obstetric registrar on call at a tertiary obstetric hospital. You have been called in to see Mrs Bryant, a 24-year-old woman at 10 weeks gestation with severe hyperemesis gravidarum of pregnancy. She has presented to the Emergency Department.

Q2

You have admitted Mrs Bryant for rehydration and investigation. The results of the tests you have ordered are as follows:

- TSH: very low
- Free T4: markedly elevated
- Thyroid receptor autoantibodies: +ve

Please advise Mrs Bryant as to your management and how the diagnosis will impact on the management of the pregnancy.

Q3

The obstetric resident calls you from the antenatal clinic to see Mrs Bryant at 36/40. Her hyperthyroidism is stable and the pregnancy has otherwise progressed well. He has just confirmed with ultrasound that the baby is a breech presentation. Please counsel the patient.

Q4

Your external cephalic version is successful, and she goes into spontaneous labour at 39/40, delivering a healthy baby girl. The midwife calls you immediately after a difficult delivery of the placenta, as Mrs Bryant has started to bleed heavily, and a lump has appeared at the introitus.

Please outline your management.

H3 Encounter 1

A 25-year-old woman, Miss P, has been referred to you for consultation. Her mother has just been diagnosed with ovarian cancer and she wants to know what her own risk is, and if anything needs to be done about it if she has increased risk.

Please take a history from Miss P.

Encounter 2

Physical examination of Miss P is unremarkable. What will you advise her regarding her risk of ovarian cancer?

Encounter 3

If the patient belongs to a hereditary breast/ovarian cancer family, what are the possible genes involved, and what is her possible lifetime risk of ovarian cancer?

Encounter 4

"What do you advise as the next step, doctor?"

Encounter 5

Miss P tests positive for BRCA1. She wants to have a family one day. What do you advise her?

H4 Encounter 1

Mrs Rajendran is a 30-year-old woman, recently migrated from India, who presents to see you in your rooms with a history of heavy menstrual bleeding. Please take a history and advise on management.

Encounter 2

The hysteroscopic resection of the submucosal fibroid proceeds without any operative complications. Mrs R is discharged from hospital the day after the operation. She is now presenting to your rooms 3 months later.

Encounter 3

Mrs R has become pregnant and has a high risk for placenta accreta on ultrasound and MRI. She is planned for an elective caesarean section tomorrow. What preparations do you instruct the obstetric resident to make?

Encounter 4

At the caesarean section a live healthy term baby is delivered. A placenta accreta is confirmed, and a caesarean-hysterectomy is performed. You are called to the post-natal ward by the midwives, who are reporting a copious watery discharge from the midline wound.

H5 Q1

Louise Waters is a 25-year-old nulliparous type I diabetic who has been referred to you for pre-pregnancy counselling.

Q2

Louise now presents to you 6 months later at 19/40 gestation. The pregnancy has been progressing well, and her BSLs are well managed in conjunction with her endocrinologist.

She has just had her 19/40 ultrasound, and the report reads:

> Singleton intrauterine pregnancy with gestation of 19/40. Normal liquor volume. No fetal anomalies identified. Placenta is anterior. Cervical os 2–3cm open, with beaking on applying pressure.

"Is my baby OK, doctor? I don't want to lose my baby!"

Q3

Describe how you would perform a McDonald cervical cerclage.

Q4

Louise is discharged after a week, without complications, with a McDonald's suture in situ. At 26/40, she presents to the Emergency Department with a watery vaginal discharge.

H6 Encounter 1

Mrs P is referred to you with a Pap smear showing a possible high-grade intraepithelial lesion. Marked inflammatory changes are also noted on the smear and organisms consistent with Candida.

Please take an appropriate history from Mrs P.

Encounter 2

Please describe your examination of Mrs P.

Encounter 3

You are seeing Mrs P a week later with the results. Here are the results:

- Pap smear: high-grade squamous intraepithelial lesions and adenocarcinoma in situ (ACIS)
- HVS: normal vaginal flora, moderate growth
- Targeted biopsy: CIN3/HPV + ACIS

Please explain the results to Mrs P.

What is your planned management?

Encounter 4
What are the potential risks of a cone biopsy?

Encounter 5
Mrs P has her cone biopsy with no complications during or immediately after the procedure. The histopathology shows CIN3/ACIS, both with clear surgical margins.

You are called to the Emergency Department as Mrs P has presented with heavy PV bleeding 12 days after her cone biopsy. The bleeding started an hour ago and she has soaked through 4 pads and is passing clots. She is feeling dizzy.

What is your management?

Encounter 6
Mrs P remains hypotensive and tachycardic and is continuing to bleed profusely, soaking through the pack you have attempted to insert in the Emergency Department.

What do you do now?

H7   ## Encounter 1
Letter
Thank you for seeing Miss C, a 28-year-old woman who presents with no periods for the past 2 years. She is recently married and wants to have a baby. Please manage her problem.

Encounter 2
The patient returns 4 weeks later for the test results. She still has not had a period and there have been no clinical changes. She is anxious for the results.

Test results
- FSH 50 IU/L & 30 IU/L one month apart
- LH 40 IU/L & 45 IU/L one month apart
- Prolactin 100 mIU/mL (0–600 mIU/L)
- TSH 2.5 (0.4–5.0)

"What do my test results show, doctor? Does anything further need to be done?"

Encounter 3
Further test results
- Karyotype 46XX
- Bone Density: T score spine −1.52, T score hip −1.6
- Vitamin D 40 (75–250)

"What do the extra tests you have ordered show?"

"Can anything be done for my hot flushes?"

"Can I have a baby in the future?"

H8 Q1

You are seeing Mrs Turnbull, a 29-year-old woman with systemic lupus erythematosus. She has been sent in by her rheumatologist for pre-pregnancy counselling as she wishes to start her family.

Please take a history and advise on your management.

Q2

Mrs Turnbull shows you the results of recent tests by her rheumatologist that you have requested:
- FBE: Hb 129, WCC 9.0, platelets 234
- Glucose tolerance test: 0 hr 4.8, 1 hr 5.7, 2 hr 5.2
- Urea and electrolytes: normal
- 24-hour urine protein/creatinine clearance: normal
- ANA: +ve
- C3/C4: normal
- Anti ds-DNA: +ve
- Anti Ro: +ve; Anti La: –ve
- Anticardiolipin antibodies: +ve

Q3

You are seeing Mrs Turnbull at 30 weeks gestation. She has just had an ultrasound and you are reading the report:
- 30/40 singleton intrauterine pregnancy
- Estimated fetal weight: 1180 g
- Moderate to severe fetal hydrops present, fetal heart rate 55 bpm
- Placenta fundal

"Is something wrong with my baby, doctor?"

6

Specialist level OSCE answers and discussion

MRANZCOG OSCE E

E1 Q1

History

- 26-year-old woman, nulliparous
- End-stage renal failure at 18 years old secondary to reflux nephropathy
- Was on haemodialysis until 23 years of age, when she received a kidney transplant from her brother
- Transplant has been reasonably successful over the last 2 years (1 episode of attempted rejection averted 3 years ago)
- Serum creatinine stable at 130 μmol/L
- Current immunosuppressive regime: Prednisolone, Azathioprine (ceased mycophenelate 18 months ago)
- Mild hypertension, controlled with atenolol
- No urinary tract infections last 12 months
- Periods 28–32 days apart, not heavy or painful; was amenorrhoeic until 6 months after transplant
- No past gynaecological history of note; uses condoms for contraception
- Last Pap smear 3 years ago, normal
- Not on folate/Elevit; has not had rubella checked
- Medical history: nil apart from above
- Surgical history: Re-implantation of ureters at 6 years old (only partially successful)
- Renal transplant surgery 3 years ago
- No family history of note
- Social Hx: Married 2 years ago, good relationship, wish to try for a baby soon
- Non-smoker, non-drinker, works in retail

5 marks

Examination

- Mild cushingoid appearance, BMI 30
- BP 130/80, PR 84, RR 12, T 37° C, urinalysis normal
- Cardiorespiratory, breast, thyroid Ex: normal
- Abdominal Ex: Scar from previous operations, otherwise normal

- Pelvic Ex (with permission): Normal-sized anteverted uterus, no adnexal masses, cervix normal on speculum Ex (can take Pap smear)

2 marks

Pre-pregnancy advice/investigations
- Pregnancy in renal transplant patients is not advisable until 2 years after transplant, due to risk of rejection, and only in transplant patients with
  - relatively normal renal function
  - no proteinuria
  - no/well-controlled arterial hypertension
  - no evidence of rejection
- Mrs Harvey should not attempt a pregnancy until she has had:
  - baseline U+E+creatinine
  - MSU – culture
  - 24-hour urinary protein and creatinine checked
  - renal/transplant physician review and involvement

2½ marks

She will need atenolol changed to metoprolol or methyl-dopa (Aldomet), as atenolol associated with IUGR and premature delivery. Not to attempt pregnancy until hypertension well controlled.

½ mark

Risks of the pregnancy, if she proceeds
Maternal
- Deterioration of renal function, graft rejection (rare – 2–5%), hypertension of pregnancy (30%), proteinuria, UTI, anaemia
Fetal
- IUGR (1/3), premature delivery (50%)

1.5 marks

Mrs Harvey should continue her immunosuppressive medications before and during the pregnancy. Normally should not take mycophenelate in pregnancy (teratogenic risk), but has already ceased it.

½ mark

- Needs rubella immunity checked
- Due for Pap smear (increased risk of cervical dysplasia with immunosuppressives)
- Needs to start Elevit/folate prior to conception

1 mark

Q2
- No change to the history
- On examination, BP 120/85, otherwise unchanged
- As long as she understands the potential risks to herself and her baby, she may start trying

1 mark

Q3

- Monthly MSU to look for bacteremia
- More frequent visits (2 weekly) to check BP and urinalysis – risk of pre-eclampsia
- Check renal function (U+E+Cr) monthly
- 24-hourly urine protein/creatinine once per trimester
- Needs glucose tolerance test (increased risk GDM on prednisolone)
- 4-weekly ultrasound for fetal biometry/growth – risk of IUGR
- Multidisciplinary management with renal transplant physician
- Should aim for vaginal delivery if possible (less risk to transplanted kidney)

1 mark for each 3 points (maximum 2 marks)

Q4

History

- 23 weeks and 3 days pregnant
- Headache for last 4 hours, not responding to Panadol
- Associated with blurry vision, and RUQ pain
- On Aldomet 500 mg QID, Labetolol 300 mg QID
- Last 24-hour urine protein 2 days ago = 1.0 g
- Renal function has been stable
- Has not had betamethasone (planned for 24 weeks)

Examination

- Drowsy, BP 170/110, urinalysis ++++protein
- Abdominal Ex: SFH=19 cm; fetal heart heard (150 bpm)
- Vaginal Ex: closed, long cervix

1 mark

Investigation/management

- Transfer to labour ward for hydralazine to control BP, and close observation
- IV access, and send off bloods:
    - FBE Hb 75, WCC 12.0, platelets 38
    - U+E+Cr creatinine 260 μmol/L
    - LFTs ALT 460, AST 320, ALP 50, albumin 30
- Patient is developing HELLP syndrome complicating severe pre-eclampsia
- She requires immediate delivery by caesarean section (likely to need classical C/S: will necessitate elective LUSCS for any future pregnancies)
- Contact haematologist – need platelets and 4–6 units of blood
- Will need general anaesthetic (not safe for spinal anaesthetic, due to thrombocytopaenia)
- Fetus is unlikely to survive given severe IUGR and severe prematurity – must counsel patient with sensitivity regarding this

- Needs hydrocortisone/steroid cover during caesarean section (long-term prednisolone)
- Will need close monitoring of renal function after delivery, in case of further decline (involve renal team)

3 marks
20 marks total

Discussion

This case requires the candidate to display a knowledge of appropriate pre-pregnancy counselling for a renal transplant patient, as well as the management of pregnancy in such a patient. Two of the most common complications in renal transplant patients are pre-eclampsia (more common in transplant patients where there is renal impairment or pre-existing hypertension, of which this patient has both), and intra-uterine growth retardation.

The candidate should be able to assess the patient in Q4 to discover severe pre-eclampsia, complicated by HELLP syndrome. The fetus must be delivered due to overwhelming risk to the mother, despite the likelihood of fetal demise. This is an emergency situation, but must still be dealt with tactfully/sensitively when counselling the mother.

E2 Encounter 1
History
- Mrs M, 62 years old
- Periods ceased at 54 years old, never used hormone therapy
- Has had several episodes of irregular vaginal bleeding over the last 3 months
- G3P3, 3 NVDs, 6 grandchildren
- Last Pap smear last year, no history of abnormal Pap smears; mammogram last year normal (has them at around same time as Pap smears)
- Hypertension, takes 2 antihypertensives (unsure what tablets she takes)
- Type 2 diabetes, treated with metformin, BSLs not well controlled. Her GP is considering changing her to insulin
- Past surgery: laparoscopic cholecystectomy, appendicectomy, right total knee joint replacement
- Strong family history of cardiovascular disease and diabetes
- Non-smoker, non-drinker; lives with her husband and loves to look after her grandchildren
- NKA medications: antihypertensives and metformin

5 marks

Encounter 2
Examination
- Obese, but otherwise well-looking
- BMI 45

- PR 96, BP 145/90
- Large abdominal pannus, skin under pannus reddened
- Vulva and vagina normal
- Speculum: blood coming through the cervical os, otherwise normal parous cervix, can take Pap smear

Investigations

- FBE
- Urea + electrolyes + creatinine
- Liver function tests
- HbA1C (glycosylated haemoglobin)
- ECG
- CXR
- Pelvic ultrasound (transvaginal)

5 marks

Encounter 3

There is an abnormally thickened endometrium for a postmenopausal woman (it should be </= 5 mm). This means that we need to perform a hysteroscopy and endometrial curettage for pathological diagnosis.

- Endometrial hyperplasia/carcinoma needs to be ruled out.
- The hysteroscopy uses either fluid or CO_2 gas to distend the potential endometrial cavity. The cavity is examined for irregular features or a polyp. Curettings are taken for histopathology and any polyps are removed.
- Risks of surgery: anaesthetic risks, infection, bleeding, perforation of the uterus (0.5%), gas embolism (rare, and only if CO_2 gas used).

Prior to surgery, will need a physician review with regards to the cardiovascular risk and diabetes. Needs a cholesterol/triglyceride check.

HbA1C is elevated at 10%. This means that for the previous 10 weeks the average glucose level was 13 mmol/L. The blood sugar levels need to be reviewed by a physician with a view to starting the patient on insulin therapy.

Serum creatinine is elevated, and need to consider diabetic renal damage (check 24-hour creatinine clearance and 24-hour protein excretion).

The patient is obese, and weight control by diet and exercise needs to be considered to decrease the associated health risks.

8 marks

Encounter 4

The patient has a cancer of the endometrium, and this will require further investigations and surgery.

- Investigations: CA125, CT scan of chest/abdomen/pelvis
- Surgery: staging laparotomy, comprising a total abdominal hysterectomy, bilateral salpingo-oophorectomy, and bilateral pelvic lymph node dissection

- Increased risk of wound breakdown and infections due to obesity, pannus and diabetes

Depending on the findings of the staging laparotomy, Mrs M may or may not require radiotherapy (either to the vaginal vault, or to the whole pelvis).

Chemotherapy is only used in advanced cases, and the tumour is not usually very responsive to it.

2 marks

20 marks total

Discussion
This represents a straightforward case of endometrial carcinoma, with the complication of obesity and poorly controlled diabetes in the patient. Diabetes and obesity are both risk factors for endometrial carcinoma.

An examination candidate at specialist level would be expected to perform well at this station.

E3 Encounter 1
The history and examination should be brief in this station (labour ward emergency).

History
- Mrs CK, 27-year-old primigravida, term singleton pregnancy
- Spontaneous onset labour 12 hours ago, SROM 3 hours ago (clear liquor)
- Fully dilated 2.5 hours ago, pushing 2 hours
- Using nitrous gas for analgesia
- NKA, No medications/IV at present
- No medical/obstetric problems
- CTG – baseline FHR 160 bpm, reduced variability, deep variable decelerations with delayed return to the baseline

Examination
- BP 140/80, PR 100, T 37°C
- Term fundus, no head palpable above the pelvic brim
- VE – fully dilated, cephalic, position OA, station 1 cm below ischial spines, moderate moulding, some caput, some descent with pushing

3 marks

- The candidate is expected to perform immediate delivery of the baby due to fetal distress and prolonged second stage. If a vacuum/ventouse is asked for, it is not available/broken.

PROMPT: "Please describe how you would perform a Neville-Barnes forceps delivery."

N.B. For both this part (performance of forceps) and station 2 (Mx of shoulder dystocia) some examinations may involve a model so that the manoeuvres can be physically demonstrated to the examiner.

- Call for assistance (senior midwife), to assess for contractions (already determined in Hx/Ex: adequate station and position, no head above the brim)

Some candidates may request a trial of forceps in the operating theatre (acceptable)

- Place patient in lithotomy, in stirrups
- Empty bladder
- Adequate analgesia: pudendal nerve block
- Apply first the left, then the right blade of the forceps, with obstetric cream for lubrication, inserting *between* contractions
- Check positioning of the blades – posterior fontanelle should be midway between the forcep blades
- Exert gentle traction in direction of the birth canal during contractions, with a maximum of three pulls/contractions. If undelivered after three pulls, failed instrumental delivery and requires immediate emergency caesarean section
- Extension of head after occiput passes under the symphysis
- Perform right mediolateral episiotomy once the head is on the perineum

4 marks

Encounter 2

The candidate is expected to run through the management of shoulder dystocia.

The baby will be delivered in good condition at the point that the candidate removes the posterior arm – until then, if the candidate asks, the baby remains undelivered.

- Call for additional help (most experienced midwifery and obstetric staff available)
- One midwife to commence documentation and call out timing at regular intervals
- Stop patient pushing
- Move patient's buttocks to the edge of the bed (bladder already empty, and episiotomy already cut from forceps delivery)
- Perform McRobert's manoeuvre (extreme flexion/abduction of the maternal hips)
- Supra-pubic pressure downward and lateral for up to 30 seconds (Rubin I)

Internal manoeuvres

1 Rubin II – push anterior shoulder from behind towards fetal chest
2 Rubin II/Woods corkscrew – use extra hand, pushing backwards on the posterior shoulder at the same time as Rubin II
3 Reverse Woods corkscrew – slide fingers from back of anterior shoulder to back of posterior shoulder and push posterior shoulder towards fetal chest

Removal of the posterior arm – move the posterior arm anterior to the fetal body, flex at the elbow, sweep the arm across the fetal chest, delivering the arm by pulling on the forearm

6 marks

Encounter 3
The history is as described in the question.

Examination
- Patient distressed, wheezing, and looking flushed
- BP 100/60, PR 110 bpm, T 38 °C

The candidate is expected to recognise a blood transfusion reaction.

Management
- Cease blood transfusion
- Give oxygen by mask
- Resuscitate with colloid (e.g. Gelafusion)
- Check label on blood and on patient
- Give IV antihistamine (Phenergan 25 mg) and 100 mg IV hydrocortisone
- Consider adrenaline in anaphylaxis/severe reaction (1 mL of 1:1000 adrenaline IM, repeated in 10 minutes if necessary)
- Contact haematology lab/haematologist

3 marks

Encounter 4
The patient is distressed due to her baby's injury. The candidate should explain the following points in a sensitive manner:
- The injury is due to stretching of the nerves of the brachial plexus during the delivery. Without effecting timely delivery of the baby, far worse injury to the baby (e.g. hypoxic brain injury) may have resulted.
- The nerve injury may take up to 6–12 months to fully resolve. However, in more than 90% of cases there is no permanent injury.
- The paediatric team will be involved in assessment/management of the baby.
- The main issue for any further pregnancies is the appropriate mode of delivery.
- The risk of shoulder dystocia in the next pregnancy is increased compared with the general population (1–16% recurrence).

The options for the patient include:
- caesarean section for future pregnancies
- attempted vaginal birth, if estimated fetal weight by ultrasound at 36/40 gestation is <4 kg. Emergency caesarean section if intrapartum risk factors for recurrent shoulder dystocia are present (e.g. slow progress of labour, need for induction of labour). Experienced accoucher to be present at the birth.

Either option is reasonable.

4 marks
20 marks total

Discussion

This station must be conducted in such a fashion as to simulate the urgency of the real-life labour ward emergencies represented.

For encounter 1, if a ventouse/vacuum is the preferred method of instrumental delivery the examiner may allow the description of a vacuum delivery. In this case, the management is the same as for forceps delivery, except:

- optimal cup placement is 3 cm anterior to the posterior fontanelle (in OA position), placed between contractions
- a check is made that no maternal tissues or vaginal wall are trapped between the cup and the baby's head
- pressure of the vacuum is gradually increased to -0.8 kg/cm^2
- once 'chignon' has developed (wait 1–2 minutes) traction is applied at right angles to fetal head, with one hand pulling the vacuum device and the other inside the introitus with one finger on the fetal head and one on the cup to monitor force of contraction and anticipate cup detachment
- again, allow only three pulls during three separate contractions
- it is not always necessary to cut an episiotomy with a vacuum delivery.

For the management described in encounter 2, the 'HELPERR' mnemonic from the Advanced Life Support in Obstetrics course may be useful:

H – Call for help
E – Evaluate for episiotomy
L – Legs (McRoberts)
P – Suprapubic pressure
E – Enter manoeuvres (internal manoeuvres)
R – Remove posterior arm
R – Roll the patient (all-fours position)

Shoulder dystocia occurs in approximately 0.6% of births, with the majority of cases not having any predisposing risk factors (e.g. fetal macrosomia, maternal diabetes, PHx shoulder dystocia, prolonged first or second stage labour, maternal obesity). All labour ward staff should reasonably be expected to know how to manage this obstetric emergency well.

Although in this case the shoulder is delivered after removal of the posterior arm, if this manoeuvre had failed the further courses of action would include repeating the internal manoeuvres with the patient rolled from the lithotomy position onto all-fours, and then manoeuvres of last resort. Manoeuvres of last resort include (in no particular order):

- Zavanelli manoeuvre – pushing the fetal head back into the birth canal and performing a caesarean section
- cleidotomy – deliberate fetal clavicular fracture by upward pressure on mid-portion
- general anaesthesia – to relax uterine muscle
- maternal symphysiotomy – dividing the maternal symphysis after a local anaesthetic.

In encounter 3, the initial management of a transfusion reaction is expected from the candidate.

In encounter 4, the candidate is expected to show concern for the mother's fears regarding the brachial plexus injury, and to gently reassure with the information in the above answer. Any reasonable approach, emphasising patient choice after carefully imparting the appropriate information regarding risk of recurrence, is acceptable. The authors accept that different approaches to mode of delivery may be employed in different obstetric units.

E4 Encounter 1

History

- Married for 5 years and ceased using the combined oral contraceptive pill 5 years ago in order to become pregnant
- 28 years old and nulliparous
- Has 28–30 day cycles and the periods last 4 days with primary dysmenorrhoea
- Her last Pap smear was 1 year ago
- No past gynaecological history of note. No past STDs/PID
- He is 28 years old and has never fathered any children
- No injuries/surgery to testes. No STDs. No past history of mumps orchitis
- Both healthy with no other personal history of note
- Sex 2–3 times a week, occasional dyspareunia
- They have no family history of note
- Non-smokers and occasionally drink alcohol. She is taking folic acid supplementation at a dose of 1 mg/day
- She is a primary school teacher and he is a secondary school teacher
- They are both very frustrated and anxious about their inability to become pregnant

5 marks

Examination

Mrs F

- Normal BP and BMI 22
- Vaginal examination shows a normal size anteverted uterus which is mobile and non-tender and there are no masses palpable, but there is some tenderness on the left side. Other examination is normal.

Mr F

- Normal pattern of body hair and a male habitus. BMI is 24.
- 20 mL testicles bilaterally which are soft and non-tender. There is no hydrocoele or varicoele and there is a palpable Vas. There are no other findings.

3 marks

Investigations
- Female hormonal profile including testing for ovarian reserve (days 2–4 FSH, LH, E_2), mid luteal progesterone and TSH
- Rubella and varicella immunity
- Semen analysis and immunobead test for antisperm antibodies

2 marks

Encounter 2
- No change to history or examination for either patient
- The candidate is expected to discuss the investigations, keeping in mind that all the tests so far are normal
- The next step is a diagnostic laparoscopy, hysteroscopy, dye studies D&C both to assess tubal patency and to look for endometriosis

2 marks

Encounter 3
The candidate is expected to discuss the findings with the couple and the options for treatment.

Treatment initially would be surgical and take place with a laparoscopic surgeon credentialed to perform grade 4 endometriosis surgery. The principles of treatment are to normalise the anatomy and to make sure that the ureter is identified and dissected.

The patient will require a bowel prep, and a bowel surgeon will need to be notified, if required.

The bowel will need to be dissected from the pouch and adhesions divided so that the left ovary is seen. The endometrioma should be removed as much as is possible and any residual cyst within the ovary diathermied. At the end of the operation the anatomy should be normalised.

Surgical excision of the endometriosis may improve the chances of natural conception.

4 marks

Encounter 4
The candidate is expected to offer treatment options and, given the severity of the endometriosis, IVF is recommended. The principles of IVF need to be known with stimulation of the ovaries to cause maturation of multiple follicles, vaginal egg retrieval (under ultrasound guidance) and fertilisation using standard IVF (rather than microinjection of the eggs) as the semen analysis is normal. Transfer of 1 embryo into the uterus 3–5 days after egg pick-up to minimise the risk of twins.

Risks of IVF to be discussed with the patients: Ovarian hyperstimulation syndrome (OHSS) and multiple pregnancy.

4 marks

20 marks total

Discussion
The candidate is expected to take a relevant history from both partners, to examine both partners, to discuss the diagnostic tests for infertility and discuss relevant treatment options, given the aetiology of the infertility.

Principles of both surgery for severe endometriosis, as well as IVF treatment are assessed in this OSCE.

E5 Encounter 1
History
- Mrs M, currently 36 weeks pregnant
- 3 previous pregnancies (6-year-old daughter, 4-year-old and 2-year-old sons)
- All deliveries were by caesarean section. The first was at 28 weeks with a breech presentation and an APH. The second two were elective and uncomplicated
- This pregnancy, persistent bleeding beginning at 23 weeks' gestation. Mrs M has been an in-patient since 23 weeks, with small vaginal blood-loss 2–3 times per week since her admission. No large bleeds
- No gestational diabetes or hypertension during this pregnancy
- Medical problems: mild asthma
- Surgical Hx: appendicectomy at 14 y.o. (open, not ruptured)
- Allergic to penicillin (facial swelling and shortness of breath)
- Interior designer, husband is a builder; supportive parents, with mother and father currently staying to help look after the 3 children at home

3 marks

Encounter 2
- FBE
- Urea, electrolytes and creatinine
- Urinalysis – looking for blood suggestive of bladder invasion
- Coagulation profile
- Group and hold, cross-match of minimum 4 units of blood
- Ultrasound of uterus + placental site
- MRI of uterus and placental site (N.B. Although often ordered, the role of MRI in diagnosing/managing placenta percreta is still to be determined)

2 marks

Anaesthetic review
- Consultation with gynaecology oncology regarding possible assistance at the time of surgery
- May also discuss with urology if possible bladder involvement
- Discuss with patient regarding:
  - risk of caesarean hysterectomy
  - risk of surgery

* transfusion (including risks of transfusion)
* damage to ureters
* damage to bladder (potential for bladder dysfunction)
* infections (lung, wound, urine, pelvis)
* need for midline incision (increased risk of herniation long-term)

2 marks

Encounter 3
• Could leave the placenta in situ and treat the patient with methotrexate.
• Could perform arterial embolisation following delivery.

2 marks

Encounter 4
1 Divide the pelvic peritoneum parallel to the infundibulopelvic ligament to enter the retroperitoneal space.
2 Identify the external iliac artery and vein laterally, and the ureter medially.
3 Retract the ureter medially to expose the common iliac artery.
4 Identify the internal iliac artery as it branches from the common iliac artery.
5 Expose the internal iliac artery. Identify the internal iliac vein as it runs below the artery.
6 Ligate it distal to the posterior division, either by:
  – using a right angle clamp to divide the tissue between the internal iliac artery and the internal iliac vein and pass a ligature around the artery. Secure this.
  OR
  – a surgical clip may be applied across the artery.
7 Care must be taken to avoid damage to the internal iliac vein.
8 Before ligating the internal iliac artery re-identify the external iliac vessels and the ureter to ensure the correct vessel is ligated.

5 marks

Encounter 5
Branches of the internal iliac artery
Anterior division
• Obturator
• Internal pudendal
• Inferior gluteal
• Umbilical
• Uterine
• Vaginal
• Middle rectal

Posterior division
- Iliolumbar
- Lateral sacral(s)
- Superior gluteal

Ligation of the posterior division may produce symptomatic ischaemia of the buttocks and sciatic nerve.

6 marks
20 marks total

Discussion

With rising caesarean section rates, the numbers of cases of placenta accreta, increta and percreta have also risen. The highest risk of placenta percreta is in a woman with multiple previous caesarean sections and an anterior low-lying placenta over the area of the previous scar. In such patients it is necessary to have a high index of suspicion, so that appropriate investigations and management are carried out. If suspected, transfer the patient to a tertiary obstetric hospital with appropriately experienced surgeons, should it occur.

E6 **Encounter 1**
History
- Mrs B, 80 years old
- Vulval pruritis for the last 30 years
- Her local doctor has prescribed Canesten cream, Ovestin cream, and a mild corticosteroid cream at various times, but none of these treatments have worked. He has never examined her.
- More recently, Mrs B has noticed bleeding from the vulva on and off, and "I can feel a lump". Bleeding is only with wiping, and associated with the lump.
- G7P4, 4 NVDs, 3 miscarriages, 10 grandchildren, 2 greatgrandchildren
- Menopause at 50 years old, no hormone therapy used
- No postmenopausal bleeding until the past 4 months
- She has never had a Pap smear, but has regular mammograms (last one last year, normal)
- No past surgical history
- Hypertension, treated with Atenolol 50 mg oral daily, well controlled
- No family history of note
- Non-smoker; drinks a glass of brandy each night before dinner, sometimes a glass of wine
- Lives with her 82-year-old husband, both fit and well, still drives, opens her bowels once per week, plays bingo on Thursday evenings

4 marks

Encounter 2
Examination
- Looks generally well
- BMI 24

- PR 84 BP 145/80
- No lymphadenopathy in neck or groin
- Chest clear
- Abdomen soft, non-tender, no masses or scars
- Vulval Ex: a 3–4 cm irregular raised ulcerated lesion on the right labia, lichen sclerosus on both labia and perineum
- Vagina atrophic
- Cervix atrophic on speculum examination (can take smear)
- PV uterus not enlarged, no adnexal masses

4 marks

Encounter 3
Investigations
- Biopsy of vulval lesion
- FBE
- Urea, electrolytes and creatinine
- Liver function tests
- APTT/INR
- ECG
- CT chest, abdomen and pelvis to look for metastatic disease and for lymphadenopathy

4 marks

Encounter 4
The patient needs to be referred to a gynaecological oncologist for definitive management.

1 mark

Encounter 5
The patient is referred because data shows that overall survival is improved with management by a gynaecological oncologist, as this is an uncommon gynaecological malignancy.

Management will be wide local excision, with 1 cm skin margins around the tumour and deep excision of tissue to the level of the deep fascia.

It is a lateral lesion, so right groin node dissection is necessary, OR sentinel lymph node procedure. (The candidate should be aware of the use of sentinel lymph node biopsy in vulvar cancer.)

Risks of surgery
Groin wound infection/necrosis/breakdown, wound seroma, deep venous thrombosis/pulmonary embolus, femoral nerve injury, chronic leg oedema/lymphangitis, stenosis of the introitus/dyspareunia/sexual problems.

If groin nodes positive, need post-operative radiotherapy to groin and pelvis.

Will need post-operative reviews for recurrence.

7 marks
20 marks total

Discussion

This patient presents with a stage II vulval SCC (tumour confined to the vulva/perineum, > 2 cm diameter, with no clinical evidence of groin node involvement). The prognosis, if treated appropriately with a gynaecological oncologist, is good, with an overall 5-year survival of 70–80%.

The candidate is expected to be aware of recent literature regarding use of sentinel lymph node dissection in the treatment of early stage vulvar cancer (Van der Zee et al. 2008). It has been reported that using radioactive tracer and blue dye to identify the sentinel groin node, groin dissection can be limited to the sentinel node only in stage I–II vulvar cancer. If the node is negative, no further groin node dissection is necessary, reducing the incidence of serious post-operative complications associated with extensive groin node dissection.

The lichen sclerosus that Mrs B has suffered from is a risk factor for the development of vulval SCC.

Reference

Van der Zee A G J, Oonk M H, De Hullu J A et al 2008 Sentinel node dissection is safe in the treatment of early-stage vulval cancer. Journal of Clinical Oncology 26:884–889

E7 Encounter 1
History

- 25 years old
- Menarche 14 years
- Regular periods until 2 years ago. Periods were every 28–30 days, lasting 5 days with no problems. For the past 2 years periods increasingly irregular, every 3–4 months and now no period for 6 months. Periods now last 5 days but often can have light bleeding for weeks at a time
- Single, sexually active for 5 years. Using condoms. Pap smear normal 6 months ago
- Acne as a teenager and has recurred in the past 2 years. Using cosmetic measures which are not helping
- Hirsutism on chin (plucks hair), around nipples (no treatment), on abdomen (waxes) and waxes legs every week. Problem has occurred over the past 2 years and is causing embarrassment. Some hair loss, which is mild, occurring on scalp generally
- No voice deepening, change to body shape, clitoral enlargement
- Now size 20. Started to gain weight 2 years ago (20 kg total weight gain). No exercise and eats poorly
- No past history – medical or surgical
- Mother has type II diabetes, father has hypertension
- No allergies, no medications, non-smoker, occasional alcohol

3 marks

Examination
- BMI 40
- BP 110/75
- Terminal hair on upper lip, chin, around nipples and thick hair over lower abdomen. Thick hair over lower arms and legs and lower back. If asks for Ferriman-Gallway score 32. Acne around chin and on shoulders
- Acanthosis nigricans on nape of neck
- Thyroid normal, no galactorrhoea
- No pink abdominal striae
- Other examination: normal, including vaginal examination

3 marks

Investigations
- FSH, LH, prolactin, testosterone, DHEAS, TSH and/or FAI, SHBG
- Pelvic ultrasound

2 marks

Encounter 2
The results show that the patient has PCOS, based on both biochemical, clinical and ultrasound evidence. Biochemical evidence shows an abnormal LH:FSH ratio, elevated T and FAI. The ultrasound shows PCO.

2 marks

PCOS is a common endocrine or hormonal disorder which can cause failure to ovulate, irregular periods, acne, unwanted hair growth, and can be associated with weight gain and insulin resistance.

2 marks

The long-term health risks of PCOS include hypercholesterolaemia/hyperlipidemia, development of diabetes, heart disease and an increased risk of endometrial hyperplasia and cancer due to elevated, unopposed estrogen levels.

The patient needs to have cholesterol/lipid levels checked, as well as be screened for diabetes (glucose tolerance test, lipid profile).

2 marks

Encounter 3
The GTT is normal and will need repeating in 2 years.

The lipid profile is abnormal (increased LDL/HDL ratio) and will need repeating in 6–12 months once lifestyle changes have occurred.

2 marks

Lifestyle changes including seeing a dietitian, and exercise either by joining a gym or in an organised exercise program.

1 mark

Treatment for Miss B's hirsutism include cosmetic measures, as well as hormonal, as it will take at least 6 months for hormone treatment to be effective.

- Cosmetic measures: shaving, depilatory creams, electrolysis
- Hormonal treatment: oral contraceptive pill with an antiandrogen (Yasmin or Diane 35) ± antiandrogen such as aldactone
  The oral contraceptive pill will have the added benefit of regulating the menstrual period.

2 marks

In the future, if she wishes to conceive, Miss B may require ovulation induction therapy such as clomiphene citrate, gonadotrophins or laparoscopic ovarian drilling ('golf-balling'), but she is not ready to start a family at present.

1 mark
20 marks total

Discussion
The expectation is that the candidate will take an adequate history such that PCOS is suspected and that the investigations are appropriate for diagnosing the problem and excluding other causes for the history. With the history it will be apparent that the patient is concerned about hirsutism and appropriate treatment will be discussed. In addition to treatment for the medical problems, as this patient is significantly overweight, lifestyle measures need to be discussed. Marks will not be awarded for investigations that are not appropriate.

E8 Q1
History
- 32-year-old primigravida at 8/40 gestation by early ultrasound
- Dizygotic twins by early ultrasound
- Planned pregnancy by IVF. Required 6 cycles to achieve pregnancy. Had a double embryo transfer for her last cycle of treatment (previously having single embryo transfers)
- Reason for IVF: male factor infertility (low sperm count)
- Mild hyperemesis gravidarum and breast tenderness
- Was on folate at time of pregnancy, and rubella immune (checked by IVF specialist)
- Has not had any antenatal testing yet
- Regular cycle 28 days, periods not heavy or painful; no intermenstrual or post-coital bleeding
- No history of STDs/PID. Last Pap smear 1 year ago (normal, always normal)
- No medical history of note
- No past surgical history
- No family history of note
- Married (good relationship). Non-smoker, non-drinker, no recreational drugs. Works as a marketing manager for a superannuation company.

4 marks

Examination
- Well-looking woman
- BP 130/65 PR 82 RR 12
- BMI 23; urinalysis normal
- Cardiorespiratory, breast, thyroid Ex: normal
- Abdominal Ex: normal
- PV/speculum: declined

1 mark

Management
- Needs routine antenatal tests ordered
- Should be on iron tablets due to increased risk of iron deficiency anaemia with twins

1 mark (½ mark each)

- Needs discussion regarding Down syndrome screening (first trimester the most accurate, as nuchal translucency of each twin allows identification of likely affected twin) – patient elects to have first trimester Down syndrome screening

1 mark

PROMPT: "Is there any way I can tell that my babies don't have Down syndrome, doctor?"

Risks of twin pregnancy need to be discussed:

Antenatal

Maternal
- Miscarriage rate increased; exaggerated general symptoms of pregnancy (e.g. backache and gastro-oesophageal reflux); APH; gestational hypertension/PET; gestational diabetes; PPROM; premature delivery

Fetal
- Congenital anomalies; IUGR; perinatal mortality; growth discordance (not associated with twin–twin transfusion syndrome)

Intrapartum
- Increased need for operative delivery (forceps, breech extraction of second twin, caesarean section), with increased risk of trauma to mother and baby

Postpartum
- PPH; breastfeeding difficulties (need supply for two babies); financial difficulties; postnatal depression (partly due to increased stressors and increased intervention needed at birth)

4 marks, depending on completeness

Plan for management of pregnancy needs to be discussed:
- Increased frequency of antenatal visits; urinalysis with each visit; glucose tolerance test at 26–28/40; fetal biometry of both twins every 4/52 after 28/40; fetal monitoring with CTG after 32/40
- Mode of delivery depends on presence of other pregnancy complications and presentation of first twin (only allow vaginal

delivery if twin 1 cephalic; if vaginal delivery, needs elective epidural, IV access, and continuous CTG monitoring, as well as delivery by experienced obstetrician)

3 marks, depending on completeness

Q2

- No change to history or examination
- High-risk result for first trimester Down screening, with twin 2 the most likely affected
- Other possibilities for increased nuchal translucency in twin 2: cardiac abnormalities, early twin–twin transfusion syndrome if chorionicity incorrect (unlikely, as early scan)
- Recommend chorionic villous sampling or amniocentesis for both twins to determine karyotype
- Will have double the risk of causing a miscarriage (i.e. 2% with CVS, 1% with amniocentesis)
- Small risk of causing damage to intervening amniotic membrane, causing an iatrogenic mono-amniotic pregnancy (high risk of cord accident and FDIU)
- Needs anti-D IgG to prevent rhesus isoimmunisation (negative blood group)

3 marks

Q3

Had CVS of both twins without complication. Currently 14/40 gestation

Options

1 Termination of both twins by either suction curette/dilatation and evacuation of uterus, or by medical termination with misoprostol vaginally. Will need anti-D.
2 Selective feticide of affected twin by intracardiac injection of **potassium** chloride, as a dizygotic pregnancy, without a shared circulation. Safe for non-affected twin (<5% unintended loss of non-affected twin), but still increased risk of premature delivery of the remaining twin.
   Can plan to deliver the remaining twin vaginally as long as cephalic presentation, and no other contra-indications to vaginal delivery.
3 Expectant management, if does not wish to undergo termination of pregnancy of either twin. Second twin has increased risk of FDIU, especially if co-existent congenital abnormalities, but FDIU of affected twin will not cause increased risk of cerebral palsy/FDIU of unaffected twin as long as no shared circulation (as appears to be the case in this patient).

3 marks
20 marks total

Discussion
The incidence of twins and triplets has increased in Australia and New Zealand with the use of assisted reproductive technologies such as IVF. The difficulty of maternal serum screening for Down syndrome in these patients is that the result is not fetus specific, and that a raised result in one twin may be masked by a normal result in the other. Therefore, the best screening test available, which is fetus specific and non-invasive, is the measurement of nuchal translucency by ultrasound in the first trimester. The addition of first trimester maternal serum screening may increase the sensitivity of nuchal translucency measurement.

The candidate in this OSCE is expected to counsel the patient about the management of a twin pregnancy, and to demonstrate an understanding of Down syndrome screening in a twin pregnancy. The second part of the OSCE tests the candidate's ability to counsel and manage a patient, first with a high-risk screening result and then with an anomalous Down syndrome dichorionic twin pregnancy.

MRANZCOG OSCE F

F1 Encounter 1
History
- Mrs K, 28 years old
- 6-month history of right iliac fossa pain and discomfort, increasing in intensity over the past 2–3 weeks
- LMP 1 week ago, very heavy period; first period in 6 months (has had an irregular cycle for the last 12 months)
- Pap smears up-to-date, never abnormal
- Nulliparous
- Past Hx: appendicectomy (aged 10); tonsillectomy
- NKA Nil medications
- No significant family history
- Works as a busy solicitor for a large corporation, travels a lot for work
- Non-smoker, occasional alcohol

4 marks

Encounter 2
- BMI 20
- BP 120/75, PR 72, RR 12
- No lymphadenopathy
- Chest clear
- Abdominal Ex: palpable tender mass in RIF, bowel sounds normal
- Vulva and vagina normal appearance
- Speculum Ex: normal cervix
- Bimanual pelvic Ex: tender mobile mass, separate from uterus, arising from the pelvis in right adnexa

3 marks

Encounter 3
- FBE, urea + electrolytes + creatinine, LFTs, coagulation profile
- Tumour markers: CA125, CA19.9, alpha-fetoprotein, LDH, inhibin, beta-HCG
- CXR
- CT scan of abdomen + pelvis
- Frozen section histology at the time of surgery

2 marks

Encounter 4
History (brief)
- Sudden onset of sharp, intense, constant pain
- Associated with nausea
- Feeling dizzy and sweaty
- No recent infections, no PV bleeding
- Bowels and bladder function normal

Examination
- BP 70/30, PR 130, RR 20
- Pale and sweaty
- Abdominal Ex: rigidity and guarding

Management
(Give results if asked for)
- FBE Hb 70, WCC 15.2; beta-HCG negative; urea + electrolytes normal
- Previous blood results not available
- Group and hold/cross-match 4 units of blood
- Commence active resuscitation/blood transfusion
- Give analgesia
- Anaesthetic review (urgent), and arrange theatre (urgent) as Mrs K has an acute abdomen
- Consent for laparotomy for suspected ruptured ovarian cyst/mass with haemorrhage
- Will require a midline incision, and consent for unilateral salpingo-oophorectomy (fertility-sparing surgery is necessary until the diagnosis is confirmed)
- Try to get frozen section histology at time of surgery (unavailable as the pathologist is ill)

5 marks

Encounter 5
The high level of inhibin raises the strong possibility of a granulosa cell tumour of the ovary.

A hysteroscopy, dilatation and curettage needs to be performed prior to definitive surgery, as approximately 75% of germ cell tumours produce oestrogen. This can cause endometrial changes ranging from hyperplasia to frank carcinoma (up to 13% risk).

The hysteroscopy should be performed prior to a staging laparotomy, as the diagnosis of an endometrial cancer may alter the surgical management.

If endometrial pathology is absent, the staging laparotomy would be as follows:

1 Midline incision.
2 Peritoneal washings for cytology.
3 Unilateral salpingo-oophorectomy (germ-cell tumours are very rarely bilateral).
4 Inspection of the other ovary, peritoneal surfaces (including diaphragm and liver capsule), and bowel. Any suspicious areas should be biopsied.
5 Unilateral pelvic lymph node dissection and para-aortic lymph node sampling.
6 Perform an infracolic omentectomy.

3 marks

Encounter 6
- Endometrial hyperplasia needs to be treated conservatively if fertility is to be preserved
- Give progestin therapy (either oral high dose, or Mirena) for 6 months, then repeat hysteroscopy/D+C
- Surgical management of the germ-cell tumour as described above
- Post-operative surveillance with pelvic examination, inhibin and oestradiol levels at each review
- Counsel the patient about the indolent nature of germ-cell tumours, so need for long-term follow-up
- Pregnancy is not contra-indicated.

3 marks
20 marks total

Discussion
The case presented is of a young, nulliparous woman with a germ-cell tumour of the ovary. The candidate is expected to display knowledge of management in both an elective and an acute presentation. Fertility preservation is important where possible in these cases, as well as an understanding of the risk to the endometrium from oestrogen-producing tumours.

A good review of the current management of granulosa-cell tumours is:

Schumer S T, Cannistra S A 2003 Granulosa cell tumor of the ovary. Journal of Clinical Oncology 21(6):1180–1189

F2 Encounter 1
History
- 16 years old
- Primary amenorrhoea
- Growth spurt at age 10; now taller than mother; 170 cm
- Breast development completed by 15 years

- Has acne. No hirsutism or other hyperandrogenic symptoms
- No galactorrhoea
- No menopausal symptoms
- No past history – medical or surgical
- No family history
- No allergies, no medications, non-smoker, occasional alcohol

4 marks

Examination
- BMI 20
- BP 110/75
- Acne on face
- Thyroid normal, no galactorrhoea
- No pink abdominal striae
- Other general examination normal
- Patient is not happy about any genital examination other than fleeting inspection of the vulva which looks normal

4 marks

Investigations ordered
- FSH, LH, estradiol, progesterone, prolactin
- Ultrasound

3 marks

Encounter 2
- The diagnosis is Mayer-Rokitansky-Kuster-Hauser syndrome (MRKH).

2 marks

Need to explain the use of vaginal dilators as the first treatment option for forming a functional vagina. 80–85% will be successful.

Vaginal dilators need to be used for 30 mins twice daily, applying moderate pressure.

An operative procedure such as McIndoe vaginoplasty is only considered if vaginal dilators are not successful. Treatment is best started when the patient is ready for sexual activity.

4 marks

Should offer to refer to patient support groups and professional counselling services if necessary.

1 mark

For childbearing in the future the only option is surrogacy using the patient's eggs and her partner's sperm with a surrogate uterus, as the patient, by virtue of her condition, lacks her own uterus, but has normal functioning ovaries.

2 marks

20 marks total

Discussion
The expectation is that the candidate will take an adequate history such that MRKH is suspected and that the investigations are appropriate

for diagnosing the problem and excluding other causes for the history. Appropriate management, including formation of a functional vagina and options for having children in the future, will need to be discussed. Marks will not be awarded for investigations that are not appropriate and this will contribute to a lower global competency score.

In the initial examination the candidate is expected to take into account the fact that the patient is 16 years old. Initial investigations need to be ordered in order to make a diagnosis. The candidate is expected to interpret the results, showing that the patient has MRKH. Then in encounter 2 the candidate is expected to discuss the future options for treatment, including a functioning vagina as well as future childbearing.

F3 Encounter 1
History

History of the presenting complaint
- Acutely unwell for last 24 hours
- Pain: central retrosternal chest pain; severity – mod severe 6–7/10; no radiations
- Associated features – worse with inspiration (true pleuritic pain), no change with position

Other symptoms
- Significant shortness of breath, even with mild exertion such as walking to the letterbox
- Fever: nil known
- Cough: nil
- Haemoptysis: nil
- Leg swelling: nil noted by patient
- Contact with unwell persons – no
- Recent 6 hrs each way car trip to attend a wedding; no overseas travel
- No significant medical/surgical history
- In particular no recent viral illnesses
- No allergies
- No medications
- No significant family history
- Casual work – waitress
- No partner – mother will be support person for labour and delivery

Pregnancy history
- Booked elsewhere
- Handheld antenatal record available if requested
- Dates certain
- Low risk T21 screening
- Normal 18 week anatomy scan
- All serology and Ix within normal limits
- (Rh+, Hep B neg, Hep C, HIV neg, Hb at booking 121, RPR neg, rubella immune, MSU no growth, normal Pap smear)

- Fetal movements noted today
  *History of pain, shortness of breath, cough, haemoptysis, travel, infection
  contacts ½ mark each (3 marks maximum)*

Examination
- Appearance: normal height and weight (if asked, no marfanoid features)
- Flushed, looks unwell, in pain
- Baseline obs: HR 120, RR 25, BP 105/50
- Pulse oximetry Sat 88% on room air
- Temp 37.8 °C
- Head and neck/thyroid: normal
- Cardiovascular: dual heart sounds, if asked, no pericardial rub, both carotid pulses present, no radio-radial delay, BP equal in both arms
- Respiratory: short of breath at rest. No wheeze, both lung fields clear throughout
- Abdominal Ex: fundus equal to dates, fetal heart auscultation +ve, normal rate and rhythm
- Vaginal Ex: omitted
- Lower limbs: no clinical evidence of a deep venous thrombosis
  *Respiratory, radial pulses, abdomen/obstetric, lower limbs ½ mark each
  (2 marks maximum)*

Differential diagnosis
- Pulmonary embolus (should be ruled out first in this case)
- Dissecting aortic aneurysm
- Atypical pneumonia
  ½ mark each (1 mark maximum)

Investigations
- Arterial blood gases
- ECG
- CXR, VQ, spiral CT
- Blood for procoagulants: FVL, Pr C/PrS, ATIII, LAC, ACL, Prothrombin gene mutation (pending)
  ½ mark each (2 marks maximum)

Encounter 2
Acute management
- Review/admission to high dependency unit/ intensive care
- Tertiary obstetric unit in conjunction with joint management with hematology/physician unit for adjustment of heparin dosing
- Oxygen – maintain maternal saturations above 90% and preferably above 95%
- Heparin – full therapeutic regime; anticipate conversion to fragmin/ clexane in a few days
- TED stockings

- Thoracic/vascular surgery notification
- Consideration of thrombolysis or embolic resection surgery
- Indicate no role for cardiotocography or celestone at this gestation

½ mark each (3 marks maximum)

Management of the remainder of the pregnancy
- Treat as HIGH RISK
- See fortnightly after discharge from hospital
- Offer all usual antenatal investigations e.g. GCT/FBE at 28 weeks, FBE/Rh antibodies at 36 weeks
- Monthly scans for fetal growth and wellbeing or earlier if clinically indicated
- Anticipate planned induction and vaginal delivery at 38+/39 wks provided obstetric parameters are appropriate

3 marks

Encounter 3
History
- 38 weeks gestation; Now stable on clexane 1.5 mg/kg daily
- No chest pain
- Good exercise tolerance
- Normal GCT/FBE/Ab screen
- Normal fetal growth and wellbeing with EFW on 50th centile last performed 2 weeks ago
- Spiral CT at 36 weeks no evidence of residual saddle embolus
- Letter from physician indicating preference for 6 months of therapeutic level anticoagulation due to the size of the original embolus

Examination
- Bp 115/75, HR RR normal
- Symphysiofundal height = 37 cm
- Longitudinal lie, cephalic presentation, 3/5 above brim
- Vaginal Ex (with consent): cervix 2 cm long, soft, mid-posterior, os closed

Management
- Admit for induction of labour
- Liaison with physician for anticoagulation
- Options cease clexane 24 hours prior to prostaglandin, or convert to IV heparin, stop heparin 6 hours before prostin or ARM. Would need to ensure protamine available
- Anaesthetic referral for discussion of anaesthetic agents/appropriateness of spinal anaesthetic
- Last dose clexane 24 hrs prior to first dose of prostaglandin of choice – candidate may choose prostin or cervidil as agent of choice provided they demonstrate familiarisation with the agent

3 marks

Encounter 4
Examination
- BP 110/75, PR 85
- Fundus 2 finger breadths above the umbilicus, boggy
- VE: clot in lower segment – further 100 mL expressed
- Oxytocin: 10 unit bolus given on the table
- 40 units in 1L requested: has not been connected
- Investigations (if requested) pre-op APPT and platelet count normal, Haemacue in recovery 8.5/dl

Management
- Ergometrine
- 40 units syntocinon over 4 hours
- Review again in 15 minutes
- On review: Scant loss, fundus firm and contracted, stable obs
- Contact physician/haematologist for plan of resumption of IV heparin/ clexane

3 marks
20 marks total

Discussion
Pulmonary embolism is one of the most common causes of maternal mortality. The diagnosis must be suspected and excluded in any pregnant woman with shortness of breath, hypoxemia and a normal CXR.

Candidates at the specialist level are expected to demonstrate a comprehensive knowledge of the principles of management during a pregnancy, including managing the labour and delivery. It is important to promptly recommence anticoagulation in a woman with a severe thromboembolic event such as the case presented in this OSCE.

F4 Q1
History
- Miss Bennett, 22-year-old sex worker
- Nulliparous
- Painless ulcer on the left labia appeared 2 days ago. No fever, vaginal discharge, or lymphadenopathy associated
- Has been a sex worker for the last 2 years
- No episodes of STDs/PID in past
- LMP 14 weeks ago
- Periods irregular 6–9 weeks apart; not heavy or painful; no intermenstrual or post-coital bleeding
- Last Pap smear 4 years ago (normal)
- Takes the combined oral contraceptive pill, but often forgets; often has sex without a condom for extra money from clients
- No past gynaecological operations
- No medical/surgical history
- No family history of note

- NKA; Nil medications
- Lives with another sex worker in a shared flat. Smokes 5–10 cigarettes/day, as well as marijuana roughly 3 times/week. Drinks alcohol only occasionally
- IV drug user – uses heroin roughly 4 times per week (never been tested for hepatitis C/HIV)

3 marks

Examination
- Thin-looking, tired; track marks on inside of arms
- BP 120/65, PR 72, RR 12, T 36.5° C
- BMI 17; urinalysis negative (urine pregnancy test unavailable if asked for)
- Cardiorespiratory/thyroid/breast Ex: normal
- Abdominal Ex: lower abdominal regular mass arising from the pelvis, 14/40 size; no hepatomegaly
- External genitalia: non-tender ulcer on left labia with pearly edge (can take swabs/skin scrapings if asked for)
- PV Ex: 14/40 sized smooth enlargement of the uterus; no adnexal masses
- Speculum Ex: normal cervix, no discharge (may take high vaginal swab, cervical swabs, Pap smear if asked for)

2 marks

Issues and management
- Consider admission to hospital for work-up
- Need to investigate for cause of ulceration (likely infective given occupation):
  - TPHA, VDRL, RPR (for syphilis)
  - Swabs for viral culture and immunofluorescence (for HSV; also dark-field microscopy for treponema)
  - HSV serology (IgG and IgM)
- Need to investigate for other sexually transmitted diseases
  - High vaginal swab (HVS)
  - Cervical swab for chlamydia/gonorrhoea PCR + culture
  - Urethral and anal swabs for culture/PCR
- Needs Pap smear

½ mark for each investigation (2½ marks maximum)

Possibility of pregnancy in this patient
- Needs quantitative βHCG and pelvic ultrasound (pelvic mass)
- (See answer to Q2 for issues/management once pregnancy confirmed)

1 mark

- Needs social worker/drug and alcohol counselling (tobacco/marijuana/heroin use)
- Offer methadone/buprenorphine program for harm minimisation
- Needs hepatitis B/C/HIV testing

½ mark each point (1½ marks maximum)

Q2

Pregnancy confirmed. Need to discuss if patient wishes to keep the pregnancy or not. (Miss Bennett wants to keep the pregnancy, and refuses to think about a termination of pregnancy.)

- Stop the oral contraceptive pill
- Needs routine antenatal testing, as well as tests for nutritional status (iron studies)
- Offer Down screening (patient declines)
- Stop smoking/drinking
- Try to change from IV heroin use to methadone (harm minimisation for mother and baby – will need management in a tertiary obstetric unit specialising in drug and alcohol problems)
- Needs case worker/social worker to assist with alternative housing/finances
- Risk of IUGR – will need serial ultrasounds for fetal biometry

3 marks

The ulceration is likely to be secondary to syphilis based on serological testing.

- Mandatory reporting to the Health Department
- Contact tracing (if possible)
- Must stop working as sex worker until confirmed it has been treated
- Needs IV benzylpenicillin or IM procaine penicillin (weekly benzathine penicillin does not cross the placenta well) – best as in-patient
- Repeat VDRL/RPR titre monthly, looking for reduction in titre with Rx
- Risk of congenital syphilis low as long as treated promptly (IUGR, corneal scarring, deafness, notched 'Hutchinson's' teeth, saddle nose, hepatosplenomegaly)

2 marks

Hep C +ve

- Need to check liver function tests once per trimester
- Stop alcohol completely to reduce liver damage
- Low risk of transmission to fetus (2%)
- Caesarean section does not reduce maternal–child transmission
- Avoid fetal scalp electrodes or instrumental delivery in labour if possible
- Breastfeeding is not contra-indicated

1½ marks

IV heroin use

- Try to change to methadone if patient willing, and explain benefits to the baby
- Risk of neonatal withdrawal after birth (will need observation in special care nursery/NICU)
- Do not use Narcan after delivery if baby needs resuscitation

1½ marks

Q3
- Likely re-activation of genital herpes/HSV infection (NB HSV +ve in test results)
- Need to perform speculum Ex/genital Ex: confirm ruptured membranes and check for vaginal ulceration (ulcers seen)

1 mark

Management
- Needs emergency caesarean section to reduce HSV transmission to newborn
- Paediatrician at delivery (risk of neonatal opiate withdrawal as outlined in answer to Q2)

1 mark
20 marks total

Discussion
The patient in this case presents with a complex series of interrelated problems: infections, drug use and social problems. Patients such as the sex worker presented in this scenario often do have multiple issues to be dealt with, and are best managed in a specialist obstetric unit adequately resourced to deal with drug and alcohol abuse in pregnancy, and the various social and medical issues associated with it.

This scenario tests the candidates' organisational ability. They need to address multiple issues and think broadly, addressing all of the biological, psychological and social problems.

F5 Encounter 1
History
- Married for 5 years and ceased using the combined oral contraceptive pill 3 years ago in order to become pregnant
- She is 32 years old and nulliparous
- Has 28–30-day cycles and the periods last 4 days and has never had a problem with her periods
- No past gynaecological history/problems/STDs/PID
- Last Pap smear was 1 year ago and normal
- He is 35 years old and has never fathered any children
- No past history of surgery or major injuries to the testes, no past STDs, no mumps orchitis in the past
- They are both healthy with no other personal history of note
- They have sex 2–3 times a week. No problems with erections/ejaculation/dyspareunia
- They have no family history of note
- They are non-smokers and occasionally drink alcohol. She is taking folic acid supplementation at a dose of 1 mg/day
- She is a primary school teacher and he is a secondary school teacher
- They are both very frustrated and anxious about their inability to become pregnant

6 marks

Examination

Mrs E
- Normal BP and BMI 22
- Vaginal examination shows a normal size anteverted uterus which is mobile and non-tender and there are no masses palpable. Other examination is normal

Mr E
- Mr E has a normal pattern of body hair and a male habitus. BMI is 24.
- He has 15 mL testicles bilaterally which are soft and non-tender. There is no hydrocoele or varicoele and there is no Vas felt on either side. There are no other findings

(N.B. The candidate must ask specifically what they are feeling for on genital examination.)

2 marks

Investigations
- Female hormonal profile including testing for ovarian reserve (days 2–4 FSH, LH, E_2), mid luteal progesterone and TSH
- Rubella and varicella immunity
- Semen analysis and immunobead test for anti-sperm antibodies

2 marks

Encounter 2
No change to history or examination.

The candidate is expected to discuss the investigations, particularly the fact that azospermia is diagnosed. The SA is repeated not less than 1 month later and the same result occurs. The candidate is expected to further investigate the reason for the azospermia and to discuss possible causes, keeping in mind that the Vas was difficult to palpate.

The candidate is expected to undertake screening for cystic fibrosis (CF), as it is associated with congenital absence of the Vas.

2 marks

The investigations needed for the male are FSH, LH, prolactin, testosterone, karyotype and CF screening and for the female elimination of possibility of CF mutation.

3 marks

Encounter 3
The results show a normal male hormone profile and karyotype. The likely diagnosis is obstructive azospermia secondary to congenital absence of the Vas.

1 mark

This couple will need IVF with microinjection. The male will require a testicular biopsy in order to retrieve sperm. Other options include donor insemination and adoption.

2 marks

As they are both carriers for the same CF mutation it is expected that the couple will be referred for genetic counselling and to discuss the possibility of preimplantation genetic diagnosis (PGD) to avoid transfer of an affected embryo.

Once fertilisation and embryo growth has occurred, PGD can be undertaken to avoid transfer of an affected embryo. The candidate needs to understand that PGD is not 100% accurate and that CVS or amniocentesis is recommended to the couple even after the transfer of an embryo that tests normal for CF on PGD testing.

2 marks

20 marks total

Discussion

The candidate is expected to take a relevant history from both partners and to examine both partners and discuss the diagnostic tests for infertility and relevant treatment options given the aetiology of the infertility.

Successful completion of this OSCE requires the candidate to understand the association between congenital absence of the Vas and the gene for cystic fibrosis. Furthermore, the candidate must be aware of the need to consider pre-implantation genetic diagnosis to avoid cystic fibrosis in the fetus.

F6   Encounter 1

History

- Georgia Melton, a 22-year-old nulliparous woman
- Recently went to her GP for her first Pap smear (overdue). She was unable to perform the smear, due to pain/discomfort
  (N.B. Candidate should ask if can speak with patient without husband present, to ask questions about sexual and relationship issues. If asked, patient will talk privately. "I am embarrassed to talk about this in front of my husband. I don't want him to think it is his fault.")
- First episode of penetrative vaginal sexual intercourse 4 years ago. Was consensual sex, but quite painful, and has been unable to have sexual intercourse since
- Has not suffered any childhood sexual abuse
- Met her husband, Greg, a 24-year-old plumber, 3 years ago, and married him 6 months ago. They have been unable to have penetrative sexual intercourse. She cannot tolerate insertion of fingers or penis in the vagina. Any attempt at penetration causes superficial pain, and muscle spasms of the vagina. Georgia cannot use tampons, and uses pads instead
- They are keen to start a family soon
- Georgia is able to orgasm via clitoral stimulation, and has a healthy libido. Has erotic dreams
- She finds her husband attractive, and they have a healthy and supportive relationship, "Greg is very understanding of my problem."

- Periods regular, every 28 days, lasting 3 days, not painful or heavy; no PCB/IMB
- No urinary Sx or vaginal discharge/STDs
- No vaginal ulcers/sores/dryness
- No medical problems
- No past surgery
- No family Hx of note
- No medication/NKA
- Lives with husband; non-smoker, non-drinker; is a policewoman

Examination
- No vaginal examination or speculum should be performed with this history
- If either is attempted, the patient is unable to tolerate it

10 marks

Encounter 2a

The candidate should speak to the patient both separately and with her husband.

An explanation of the condition and its cause should be delivered with sensitivity and compassion. Following that, a description of the possible modes of management should be given.

Sample answer

The patient has a condition called 'vaginismus'. It is uncommon, affecting only around 2% of the population. It consists of psychological conditioned reflex in the pelvic musculature, with muscle spasm occurring during attempts at vaginal penetration, making it difficult or impossible. Vaginismus may be triggered by an early painful sexual experience or by childhood sexual abuse.

Women with vaginismus in isolation do not necessarily have problems with libido or arousal. They may have associated issues relating to self-esteem and depression.

Fortunately, vaginismus is a treatable condition with a high chance of success, although treatment may take some time (often months or years). Treatment should be undertaken only by an experienced sexual therapist. This may involve a multi-disciplinary team including a psychologist, psychiatrist, gynaecologist, sexual therapist and relationship counsellor, or combination thereof. Some hospitals have specialist clinics to deal with these problems.

Some couples will benefit from group or couples therapy, or from patient support groups.

Treatment can be psychodynamic or psychotherapeutic, exploring the woman's feelings and improving understanding of her perception of pain. This is a lengthy treatment, but deals with the root cause.

Alternatively, physical treatment with a series of phallus-shaped devices of slowly increased diameter may be employed. These allow the woman to have control of penetration, and slowly over time allow her to get used to devices of increasing diameter. At first, the woman should engage in these exercises alone, but once more comfortable, her partner may be included in the exercises.

Success rates with both treatments approaches 90–95%.

Surgery is contraindicated as it is of no value in treatment.

Must consider strain on the relationship during treatment, and consider regular counselling for both the patient and her husband.

7 marks

Encounter 2b

With patience there is a high chance of penetrative vaginal intercourse being possible after several months of treatment.

If wishing to conceive earlier, patient has the option of the husband ejaculating on the external genitals (some chance of conception), or inseminating the patient with sperm in a syringe (usually possible except in the most severe cases).

Rarely a place for IVF in this situation – occasionally for women with failed treatment for vaginismus (will need sedation/general anaesthetic for embryo transfers), or in women with age-related fertility decline who cannot afford to wait months/years for vaginismus treatments to work.

3 marks
20 marks total

Discussion

This is a difficult OSCE for the exam candidate, but tests the recognition of and knowledge about vaginismus. It is also a good station to assess a candidate's counselling ability. Vaginismus may be uncommon but will be seen in most general gynaecology practices, especially if a high clinical index of suspicion is maintained.

F7 Q1

History

- 25-year-old primigravida, 8/40 by dates
- Spontaneous, unplanned pregnancy (but wanted)
- Was not on folate prior to conception, and rubella not checked
- Mild morning sickness and breast tenderness; no other symptoms of note
- No antenatal investigations performed yet
- Rheumatic fever as a child, with subsequent development of rheumatic heart disease, and mitral stenosis
- Had percutaneous mitral balloon valvotomy at 16 years old due to worsening symptoms, with subsequent reasonable exercise tolerance
- She currently gets breathless and tired if she climbs a single flight of stairs, but can walk long distances on flat ground without any problems. No paroxysmal nocturnal dyspnoea (sleeps on 2 thin pillows). No palpitations or chest pain

- Last echocardiogram showed a valve area of 3.0 cm^2
- Has a cardiologist, whom she last saw 9 months ago, and said she was 'stable'
- No other medical history of note
- Other than valvotomy, no other surgery
- No gynaecological history of note; last Pap smear 3 years ago (normal)
- No family Hx of note
- Non-smoker, moderate alcohol (stopped drinking once found out she was pregnant)
- Lives with husband, works as a receptionist
- NKA, No medications

3 marks

Examination
- Well-looking woman, BMI 19, no cyanosis
- Vitals: BP 110/65, PR 96 regular, T 37, RR 18
- Cardiac: Late diastolic murmur
- Respiratory: mild crackles in lung bases
- Abdominal Ex: normal
- PV/speculum: 8/40 sized anteverted uterus, no adnexal masses, normal cervix (can take Pap smear)

2 marks

Management
- Needs Pap smear
- Needs routine antenatal investigations + to be offered Down syndrome screening (patient declines the latter)
- Pregnancy needs to be managed at a tertiary hospital with both cardiology and materno-fetal medical services
- Should have an anaesthetic review prior to delivery
- Will need multi-disciplinary management with cardiology, and will need to have an echocardiogram for examination of the maternal heart once per trimester. If signs of decompensation/pulmonary oedema, will be managed in conjunction with cardiology
- No extra risk above normal of cardiac anomalies in the fetus (mother has an acquired rather than a congenital heart problem)
- Will need antibiotic prophylaxis during any invasive procedures, as well as after delivery (risk of bacterial endocarditis)

3 marks

PROMPT: "Is there anything special that will have to be done at my delivery?"
- During delivery will need to avoid fluid overload, as well as severe maternal tachycardia, as may lead to pulmonary oedema
- Vaginal delivery acceptable, as long as mother is cardiac-monitored (preferably in a cardiac unit). Needs IV access. Needs continuous CTG monitoring. Epidural anaesthesia may reduce risk of tachycardia response to pain

- Biggest risk to mother is in the second stage, and immediately after delivery
- Avoid prolonged pushing (low threshold for instrumental delivery if vaginal birth)

2 marks

Q2
History
- Fully dilated on vaginal examination 20 minutes ago. Has been pushing for 10 minutes. Acute onset of breathlessness and altered conscious state. Cardiac monitor shows an irregular heart beat consistent with atrial fibrillation. CTG monitor shows late decelerations
- Has epidural anaesthesia (working well), and IV access

1 mark

Examination
- Drowsy, non-responsive; laboured breathing
- PR 120 irregular (atrial fibrillation), BP 120/60, O2 saturation 80% (room air)
- Lungs: diffuse crackles throughout both lung fields
- VE: fully dilated, OA position, cephalic presentation, station +1 cm

1 mark

Management
- Has pulmonary oedema secondary to atrial fibrillation +/- fluid overload
- Also has fetal distress, possibly secondary to maternal hypoxia
- Maternal and fetal management needs to be concurrent, but maternal management better served by prompt delivery of the fetus
- Call for help (including cardiologist/anaesthetist/paediatrician/midwife)
- Need ventouse or forceps delivery of fetus
- Mother needs O_2 by mask + IDC (to monitor urine output)
- IV frusemide 20–40 mg bolus
- Reversion of atrial fibrillation (digoxin or direct current conversion after delivery of fetus) or rate control with beta-blockers
- May need invasive cardiac monitoring if fails to respond to medical management of pulmonary oedema

3 marks

Q3
Ninety per cent of the general population is Kell-negative. To have developed antibodies to Kell, Mrs Brock must be Kell-antigen negative. Her fetus will only be at risk if it is Kell-antigen positive.

First step is to test her husband. If he is Kell-antigen negative (90% chance), her pregnancies are not at risk.

If her husband is Kell-antigen positive, any subsequent pregnancies must be carefully monitored.

2 marks

Antibody titres do not correlate with the severity of the condition for the fetus.

Kell antibodies cause suppression of erythropoiesis, not haemolysis, so amniocentesis for optical density/bilirubin measurements are not helpful. It may be helpful for DNA testing of fetus for Kell-antigen expression, if available.

Serial antenatal ultrasound to look for signs of fetal hydrops, and measurement of middle cerebral artery resistance can be performed, with cordocentesis/fetal blood sampling if there is a suspicion of effects on the fetus.

3 marks
20 marks total

Discussion
Rheumatic heart disease is the most common heart disease in pregnancy, with the mitral valve being the most common heart valve to be involved (90% of rheumatic valvular cases). Patients with mitral valve stenosis should have their valve area assessed prior to pregnancy, and their cardiac function assessed by echocardiography. Atrial fibrillation increases the risk of the pregnancy to the patient, and should be corrected if possible prior to pregnancy.

In this case the patient presents already pregnant, but in a stable condition. The candidate is expected to outline their antenatal and intra-partum management plan for the patient, and then to manage the acute onset of pulmonary oedema secondary to atrial fibrillation during the second stage of labour. The third encounter requires the candidate to demonstrate knowledge of the management of anti-Kell antibodies with respect to pregnancy.

F8 Q1
History
- 16 years old
- Primary amenorrhoea
- Growth spurt at age 10; now taller than mother; 175 cm
- Breast development now complete
- Sparse pubic and axillary hair
- No menopausal symptoms
- No past history – medical or surgical
- No family history
- No allergies, no medications, non-smoker, occasional alcohol

2½ marks depending on completeness

Examination
- BMI 20
- BP 110/75
- Thyroid normal, no galactorrhoea
- Normal-looking breasts
- Very little axillary and pubic hair

- No pink abdominal striae
- Bilateral masses in both inguinal areas
- Other general examination normal
- Patient is not happy about any genital examination other than fleeting inspection of the vulva which looks normal

2½ marks depending on completeness

Investigations
- FSH, LH, prolactin, testosterone, estradiol, DHEAS, progesterone
- Ultrasound
- Karyotype

2 marks depending on completeness

Q2
The test results show that the patient has androgen insensitivity syndrome (AIS).

1 mark

First, the disorder needs to be explained to the patient carefully and sensitively.

A sample explanation
"You were born with a condition known as androgen insensitivity syndrome. This means that you are a woman born with 46XY chromosomes (normally male), rather than 46XX chromosomes (normally female). Because of an abnormal androgen receptor, the normal hormonal signalling that would have led to you developing into a male was switched off, so that you developed into a woman instead. A woman with AIS has normal external genitals, but lacks a uterus or ovaries as the gonads produce a hormone called anti-Mullerian hormone, which causes the embryological structures normally destined to become the uterus and upper vagina to disappear. The gonads are not ovaries, but abnormal testes which usually lie in the abdomen or in the inguinal canal."

4 marks

The gonads are abnormal due to their prolonged presence inside the abdominal cavity (or, in this case, the inguinal canals). There is a significant risk of them developing gonadoblastomas/seminomas in later life if they are not removed. The risk of tumours is 25–30% in adulthood (rarely occurs before puberty). Miss T will need excision of the gonads, which, on examination, appear to be in the inguinal canals, with a bilateral inguinal hernia repair at the same time, if required.

2 marks

Once the gonads have been removed Miss T will require long-term hormone therapy with estrogen alone (does not need progesterone as there is no uterus). The estrogen will sustain breast development and prevent osteoporosis.

2 marks

The vagina is usually functional as the lower two-thirds are well developed. If the vagina is found by the patient to be too shortened, it can almost always be lengthened with the use of vaginal dilators. Surgical vaginoplasty is only required in a minority of cases.

1 mark

Adoption is the only option for future child-bearing as the patient lacks both a uterus and ovaries. In some states/countries there may be the option for a baby with donor eggs using a surrogate mother, but there is no option for children with a genetic contribution from the patient with AIS, as she has no oocytes. This last point needs to be conveyed with tact and sensitivity.

2 marks

Should offer counselling from an experienced counsellor.

½ mark

Offer to direct the patient and her mother to patient support groups, such as the Androgen Insensitivity Syndrome Support Group (AISSG), as they can provide information and support.

½ mark
20 marks total

Discussion

In the first encounter the candidate is expected to take an adequate history, as well as perform an examination, taking into account that the patient is 16 years old. Initial investigations need to be ordered so that a diagnosis can be made.

The expectation is that the candidate will take an adequate history such that AIS is suspected and that the investigations are appropriate for diagnosing the problem and excluding other causes for the history. Appropriate management, including open discussion of the implications with the patient, the use of hormone therapy, removal of gonads and future childbearing, needs to be addressed. Marks will not be awarded for investigations that are not appropriate. The second encounter requires a lot of time spent counselling about the implications of the diagnosis.

MRANZCOG OSCE G

G1 Q1

History

- 33-year-old primigravida, 18/40 by sure dates; planned spontaneous pregnancy
- Was having routine fetal anomaly scan today
- Is booked in at the hospital antenatal clinic
- Routine antenatal investigations on antenatal card:
  - Blood group: O neg, no antibodies
  - FBE: Hb 136; MCV 88; platelets 269
  - Rubella: non-immune
  - TPHA: negative

- HepB/HIV serology: negative
- MSU: no growth
- No problems with pregnancy up until now; no fetal movements felt yet
- No medical problems
- No past surgery
- No history of recent illness/rash/fever
- Periods normal and regular, no gynaecological illness, Pap smear 6/12 ago normal
- NKA, nil medications (ceased folate 4/52 ago)
- Non-smoker, non-drinker, lives with husband (good relationship), childcare worker

3 marks

Examination
- Well-looking, no rashes, BMI 26
- BP 120/70, PR 80, T 36.5, RR 16
- Urinalysis negative
- Cardiorespiratory, thyroid, breast Ex: normal
- Abdominal Ex: 18/40 fundus, no hepatosplenomegaly
- PV: patient declines

2 marks

Management
- Patient has fetal hydrops, but no clear cause on history or examination. A thorough investigation for causes of fetal hydrops needs to be performed.
- Will need referral to the fetal diagnostic unit, materno-fetal medicine unit, or equivalent, preferably the next day.

1 mark

Investigations include
- Haemoglobin electrophoresis
- HbA1C/glycosylated haemoglobin
- Liver function tests
- Kleihauer test
- Repeat blood group and antibodies
- Serology for parvovirus, rubella, CMV, hepatitis B, toxoplasma
- Repeat ultrasound in the tertiary unit (i.e. COGU scan) to examine for fetal anomalies, especially looking at the fetal heart
- Amniocentesis for karyotype and culture

3 marks (½ mark for each correct investigation)

- Mrs White is non-immune for rubella, and will need vaccination after delivery (cannot give vaccine during pregnancy).

1 mark

- She is also Rhesus negative and will need anti-D at the time of her amniocentesis and after delivery.

1 mark

Q2

No change on history or examination.

The results show that the likely cause of the fetal hydrops is a parvovirus infection. It is likely that Mrs White has been into contact with a child with 'slapped cheek syndrome', even though there is no clear history of exposure.

Parvovirus infection causes anaemia in the fetus by suppression of erythropoiesis, and subsequent cardiac failure due to anaemia.

While 33% of cases of fetal hydrops will spontaneously recover, 33% will undergo rapid demise, and 33% will be rescued with intra-uterine blood transfusions to the fetus.

2 marks

Mrs White needs urgent fetal blood sampling via cordocentesis in the tertiary fetal diagnostic unit, as her fetus already has hydrops. Fetal haemoglobin and platelet count need to be assessed, and a blood transfusion of O negative blood (20–30 mL aliquots) to the fetus given in utero if moderate to severe anaemia is found. The fetus will need to be immobilised with a trans-uterine injection of pancuronium beforehand, and anti-D will need to be given to Mrs White to prevent possible isoimmunisation.

2 marks

Q3

- Patient is haemodynamically stable and under a general anaesthetic.
- Needs a laparoscopy to examine the internal organs for damage, and inspect the suspected perforation site.

2 marks

Q4

- Feeling well. Passing urine and faeces.
- Haemodynamically stable on examination. Afebrile. Abdomen soft.

1 mark

- Need to counsel Mrs White about the perforation.
- Will need to have elective caesarean sections for subsequent pregnancies due to risk of uterine rupture from the fundal perforation.

2 marks
20 marks total

Discussion

The causes of fetal hydrops include:

1 Immune hydrops (<10%) – Rhesus et al isoimmunisation
2 Non-immune hydrops (90%)
    - Cardiovascular (arrhythmias, congenital heart block/anti-Ro + anti-La antibodies, myocarditis, structural anomalies)
    - Other malformations – cystic hygroma, bone defects, diaphragmatic hernia, severe spina bifida
    - Aneuploidies
    - Haematological – α thalassemia, chronic abruption

- Maternal diabetes, liver dysfunction
- Twin–twin transfusion syndrome
- Infections (TORCH, especially parvovirus).

The required investigations reflect these potential causes.

The candidate is expected to show knowledge of the investigation and management of a proven maternal parvovirus infection in pregnancy. Subsequently, they are expected to manage a complication of a dilatation and evacuation of the uterus after an FDIU.

G2 Encounter 1
History
- Last menstrual period 2/52 ago; regular cycles, no intermenstrual bleeding
- Not sexually active
- Pain commenced 24 hours ago. Gradually increasing in severity, requiring pethidine
- Has noticed a gradual increase in abdominal girth over the last few months
- Short of breath on exertion
- No significant past medical history
- No allergies

Examination
- BP 110/70, PR 102, RR 18, Temp 37°C
- Abdominal Ex: large abdominal mass to level of 2 cm above the umbilicus; generalised abdominal tenderness
- Chest Ex: dull to percussion in both bases
- No lymphadenopathy
- Rectal examination declined

3 marks

Encounter 2
- FBE
- U+E+Cr
- LFTs
- Coagulation profile
- CXR
- CT scan abdomen/pelvis
- (Ultrasound not available)
- Tumour markers – beta-HCG, LDH, CA125, CA19.9, CEA, AFP

4 marks

Encounter 3
Discuss the possible diagnosis with sensitivity. Given the size and CT appearance, it is most likely benign, but there is a chance it could be a borderline or even malignant tumour of the ovary.

Miss M needs a laparotomy (midline), and either an ovarian-cystectomy or an oophorectomy.

Would like to have frozen section histology available at the time of surgery (not available at the country hospital).

Spillage of cyst contents needs to be avoided in case of malignancy.

Consent the patient, explaining risks of surgery (infection, bleeding, bowel damage if adherent to mass, possible need for removal of the ovary).

3 marks

Encounter 4

No further surgery is required. Stage 1 borderline serous tumours of the ovary have only an 8% recurrence rate, and all recurrences are usually confined to the ovary and curable.

Miss M needs monitoring with 6-monthly ultrasound and CA125 levels (if CA125 elevated with original tumour, and in this case, when the result came back it was elevated).

Consider the combined oral contraceptive pill.

3 marks

Encounter 5
History
- Vague discomfort in the right iliac fossa
- Regular menstrual cycle, no intermenstrual or post-coital bleeding
- Now sexually active, using condoms

Examination
- Normal baseline observations
- Chest clear
- No lymphadenopathy
- Abdomen: midline scar to above the umbilicus; tender RIF
- Bimanual examination: anteverted uterus, L adnexa normal, fullness and tenderness in right adnexal region with some mobility

Investigations
- Ultrasound: simple 5 cm cyst on right ovary
- CA125: normal

Management
Given patient's past history, size of cyst and symptoms, repeat surgery is recommended.

5 marks

Options for surgery include:
- open laparotomy via previous midline incision
- laparoscopic surgery (ovarian cystectomy, avoiding spillage of cyst contents) with Hassan entry given previous surgery, or possible entry with 5 mm laparoscope at Palmer's point.

2 marks

20 marks total

Discussion

The case tests the candidate's understanding of the management of a borderline serous tumour in a young girl. The emphasis in this case is on initial conservative surgery, and no need for further surgery after removal of the first tumour. The candidate is directed to the paper by Lim-Tan et al (1988), which advocates conservative management of serous borderline ovarian tumours.

Conservative management is essential to maintaining the girl's future fertility. Note that it is inappropriate to perform a vaginal examination on the patient as she is not sexually active at her first presentation.

Reference
Lim-Tan S K, Cajigas H E, Scully R E 1988 Ovarian cystectomy for serous borderline tumors: a follow-up study of 35 cases. Obstetrics and Gynecology 72(5):775–781

G3 Encounter 1

While still on growth hormone beginning at about age 10 years, very low dose oestrogen will be started. A typical regimen is 6.25µg E patch weekly with an increase in dose every 6–9 months.

The increase in the dose will depend on breast development as well as continuing use of growth hormone. E and GH together will work synergistically to increase height. Too high a dose of E with GH will negate the effect of the GH.

A baseline ultrasound needs to be performed prior to treatment, then is performed on a yearly to two-yearly basis to look at the growth of the uterus. Once an adult-size uterus is formed and there is endometrial thickness above 5 mm, progestagen can be added to the E regimen. It is expected that at this stage the dose of E will be 50 µg weekly. The P can be added in a sequential regimen to cause a withdrawal bleed. It may be 2–4 years from the time that the hormone therapy starts to a withdrawal bleed. The growth of an adult uterus is important for the ability to carry a pregnancy successfully into the future.

4 marks

Encounter 2

There are many possible health problems associated with Turner's syndrome, including:
- cardiac – (bicuspid aortic valve, aortic root dilatation) 50% risk
- renal abnormalities (duplex system/horseshoe kidney) 20% risk
- hypertension
- hypothyroidism (usually auto-immune Hashimoto's throiditis)
- deafness (recurrent otitis media)
- coeliac disease
- inflammatory bowel disease
- abnormal LFTs (15–20%)

- juvenile rheumatoid arthritis
- osteoporosis (if insufficient estrogen therapy)

4 marks

Annually the patient requires:
- FBE, U+E, creatinine, TSH, LFTs, fasting glucose and lipids, vitamin D
- ECG, echocardiogram if previously abnormal, MRI if aortic root dilatation
- MSU if previously abnormal

Every 2 years:
- Creatinine clearance, celiac antibody testing, DEXA if osteopaenia on initial examination at 21 years of age

Every 5 years:
- ECG, echocardiogram (if previously normal), DEXA if normal BMD initially, audiology 2 yearly or 3–5-yearly if normal audiology initially

4 marks

Encounter 3
- IVF with donor eggs
- Fostering
- Adoption

2 marks

Potential pregnancy problems in Turner's syndrome:
- IUGR (small uterus)
- Increased need for caesarean section (increased cephalo-pelvic disproportion)
- Dissection of aorta (aortic root dilatation plus hypertension)
- If valve abnormalities, needs antibiotic prophylaxis
- Increased risk of GDM and pre-eclampsia

2 marks

Prior to pregnancy
- MRI, cardiologist review mandatory, FBE, U+E, creatinine, creatinine clearance, MSU, vaginal ultrasound, TSH, FreeT4, thyroid antibodies, LFTs, coeliac antibodies, fasting glucose.

2 marks

Encounter 4
- If 45X/46XX mosaic, more likely to have spontaneous puberty/pregnancy, with longer preservation of ovarian function
- If 45X/46XY mosaic, 5–30% risk of dysgerminoma if leave gonads in, so need to excise them laparoscopically

1 mark each
20 marks total

Discussion

The expectation is that the candidate will be able to describe the development of secondary sexual characteristics using hormone therapy, including development of the uterus. It is also expected that they will be able to explain the long-term consequences of Turner's syndrome and explain the need for regular monitoring. The candidate should also be able to discuss future fertility options, and the pregnancy risks associated with women who have Turner's syndrome. The candidate is not expected to take a history in this OSCE, but to inform and counsel the mother regarding Turner's syndrome.

G4   Encounter 1

History

- Mrs Cook, 28 years old
- Spontaneous planned singleton pregnancy; first pregnancy
- 26/40 by dates and 12/40 ultrasound
- No problems with the pregnancy until now
- Presented to GP with headaches and blurry vision, no abdominal pain or PV bleeding
- No relevant gynae history, Pap smear 1 year ago (normal, always normal)
- Family Hx: Mother had hypertension in her pregnancies, no diabetes or other problems
- Lives with husband, non-smoker, non-drinker
- NKA, meds as above (was on folate earlier in pregnancy)

Examination

- BP 190/110, PR 80, T 37°C
- BMI 20, urinalysis = 3+ protein
- Neurological Ex: normal, no clonus or hyperreflexia
- Abdominal Ex: no RUQ tenderness, fundal height 26 cm, longitudinal lie, breech presentation, FH 140 bpm

Investigations (if asked for)

- FBE Hb 120, WCC 8.5, platelets 240
- U&E+creatinine all normal
- LFTs normal, apart from Alk Phos 120 (normal range 5–40)
- 24-hour urinary protein – 4 gm/24 hours
- Too early for CTG
- Ultrasound: Single fetus, breech presentation, 26/40 size on growth parameters, placenta anterior and fundal

Management

- Admit the patient and start arranging transfer to nearest tertiary facility
- Start IV hydralazine (5 mg aliquots until BP settles, then may start hydralazine infusion as needed)
- Give betamethasone 11.4 mg IM, with second dose 24 hours later (in case needs earlier delivery)

7 marks

Encounter 2
History and examination
- Patient distressed, breathless, and semi-conscious
- BP 160/100, PR 100, RR 28, T 37 °C
- Oxygen saturation 80%
- Patient coughing with pink frothy sputum
- Diffuse crepitations on chest auscultation, with elevated JVP
- FHR confirmed at 80 bpm

Management
- Patient going into cardiac failure
- Need to call for help from anaesthetist/intensivist/physician
- O_2 by mask until able to intubate to manage airway/ventilation
- IV Frusemide
- Need to reduce blood pressure with IV antihypertensives
- Transfer to ICU
- Patient too unwell to consider caesarean section/delivery

3 marks

Encounter 3
The BP will only be effectively controlled after delivery of the products of pregnancy. The patient is too unstable and the anaesthetists are not happy for her to undergo a caesarean section.

The patient is too unwell to be transferred by air ambulance to a tertiary centre.

The patient requires delivery vaginally by administration of vaginal prostaglandins (Prostin 2 mg PV, then 1 mg PV 12 hours later; can continue with 1 mg PV BD until delivery).

2 marks

Encounter 4
- Reassessment of patient's condition
- Patient still on ventilator, with high pressures required due to pulmonary oedema
- BP 170/100 on IV nitroprusside infusion
- VE – cervix long, hard and closed
- FBE Hb 100, WCC 13.0, platelets 56, some haemolysis
- U&E+creatinine normal
- APTT/INR normal
- LFTs starting to elevate (AST 200, γGT 250, ALP 200)
- The patient is starting to develop HELLP syndrome, complicating her severe pre-eclampsia
- Need to consider LUSCS to remove the FDIU and placental tissue, with following special conditions:
  - 4 units X-matched blood (increased risk of bleeding)
  - platelet transfusion (with advice of haematologist)

4 marks

Encounter 5
Examination/investigation

- Cyanosed, unconscious
- PR 120, BP 60/20, RR 32, O_2 saturation 70%
- Raised JVP and right ventricular heave
- V/Q scan or spiral arterial CT scan – massive pulmonary embolus
- Call medical code
- O_2 by mask; IV access
- Supportive treatment until definitive diagnosis and management can occur
- Need vascular surgeon to remove saddle embolus

4 marks
20 marks total

Discussion

In this OSCE station it is essential for the candidate to remember to reassess the clinical picture with a brief history and examination at each encounter. In encounter 2, for example, the left ventricular failure as a result of the severe PET may be missed without asking for a reassessment of the patient's condition. The history and examination must be taken in an efficient manner if the candidate is to complete all of the encounters for this OSCE.

The candidates must read all the information given. Being in a provincial hospital a case such as this should be transferred to a tertiary facility, but the patient needs to be stabilised prior to transfer. The baby must be considered as well as the patient (by performing an ultrasound, as well as administering steroids for lung maturation). However, where both mother and baby are in danger, as in this case with cardiac failure, the mother's condition must be managed and stabilised first, even if it poses a risk to the fetus.

The examiner must move the candidate quickly through the encounters in this OSCE for all of the encounters to be completed.

If this patient wishes to attempt another pregnancy, there are multiple issues including:

- the need to test for potential causes of DVT/PE and early-onset pre-eclampsia (antiphospholipid syndrome, and other thrombophilias)
- an increased risk of pre-eclampsia in next pregnancy
- an increased risk of DVT/pulmonary embolus (consider aspirin and heparin/clexane prophylaxis in next pregnancy or post-partum)
- the need to assess cardiac function with cardiologist prior to considering another pregnancy (Echocardiogram, LV ejection fraction on nuclear medicine scan)
- having had a caesarean section, her suitability for VBAC or repeat elective caesarean section must be assessed
- routine issues: rubella status, folate supplementation.

G5 **Encounter 1**
History
- 55 years old
- 3 pregnancies and 3 children born by vaginal delivery. Healthy children.
- No periods for 12 months. Prior to that about every 1–3 months for 2 years and prior to that regular
- Hot flushes and night sweats for the past 18 months. Getting worse. Difficulty sleeping, tired, irritable. Vaginal dryness and pain with intercourse
- Only had 1 partner. Used condoms in the past
- No past history, medical or surgical
- Has a glass of milk daily, no exercise, little sun exposure as works on permanent nightshift as a nurse
- Family history: mother developed breast cancer at age of 54 years
- No allergies, no medications, non-smoker, occasional alcohol
- Pap smear 6 months ago; mammogram 6 months ago – normal

5 marks

Examination
- BMI 27
- BP 120/80
- Breast Ex: normal with no masses
- General Ex: normal
- Vaginal Ex: bulky AV uterus. No masses in adnexae and no tenderness. Vaginal dryness, no evidence of major prolapse or descent

3 marks

Investigations
- Bone density
- Vitamin D

2 marks

Encounter 2
- The bone density scan shows moderate bone loss in combination with low vitamin D level
- General lifestyle changes are important to minimise lifestyle-associated decreases in bone loss, including:
  - adequate calcium intake of 1500 mg/day best obtained by dairy intake
  - 30 mins weight-bearing exercise per day
  - vitamin D intake with replacement of vitamin D and retesting in 3 months to ensure adequate replacement
  - adequate exercise will help with weight loss.

5 marks

Encounter 3
- Discuss the use of HT, including the benefits and risks, particularly with regard to the patient's own risk factors.

Benefits
- Effective relief of symptoms including vaginal symptoms
- Bone protection and treatment for osteopaenia and osteoporosis
- May protect against bowel cancer

Risks
- Deep venous thrombosis
- After 5 years slight increase in breast cancer, heart attack and stroke

3 marks

The use of HT generally is for short-term use to treat symptoms. It is expected that the use would be for 3 years initially and the patient would then cease treatment to see what happens to her symptoms.

The patient's own risks for treatment include her weight, which increases her risks for breast cancer as well as for heart disease, as well as her family history of heart disease. There is also evidence that a low vitamin D is associated with both heart disease and breast cancer.

2 marks

20 marks total (subtract 2 marks if unnecessary hormone tests are ordered)

Discussion
The candidate is expected to take an adequate history of the patient's menopausal problem and discuss HT, bearing in mind the overall risks of treatment as well as the patient's risks for the use of HT. The candidate is also expected to discuss lifestyle issues with the patient, including weight loss, adequate calcium intake and exercise. No hormone investigations need be undertaken and if they are the candidate will lose marks from their total score.

G6 Encounter 1
History
- Mrs KL, 32-year-old nulliparous woman
- Menarche 14 years old. Periods 4 weeks apart, bleeds for 4 days (not heavy), severe period pain (bedridden for 2 days each period); has tried NSAIDs with no benefit
- Associated deep dyspareunia
- LMP 1 week ago. Occasional intermenstrual bleeding, but no post-coital bleeds.
- Sexually active (married 3 months ago), not on contraception (would be happy to be pregnant, but not actively trying); no vaginal discharge
- Last Pap smear 5 years ago (always normal)
- No past gynae or medical history
- Past surgical history: appendicectomy at 16 years old (ruptured, required midline laparotomy); tonsillectomy as child
- No family history of note

- Lives with husband, good relationship; smokes 10 cigarettes per day; social drinker; works as teacher's aid
- NKA; nil medications

Examination
- Normal general appearance
- PR 72 bpm, BP120/80, T 37, BMI 20, urinalysis normal
- Cardiorespiratory, breast, thyroid Ex: normal
- Abdominal Ex: midline laparotomy scar, mild lower pelvic tenderness
- Normal vulva; normal cervix on speculum Ex (Pap smear and/or cervical swabs can be taken)
- Bimanual pelvic Ex: generalised mild tenderness
- Vaginal/rectal Ex: thickening in Pouch of Douglas

Investigations/management
- Normal STD swabs and Pap smear
- Pelvic ultrasound normal
- Discuss need for exclusion of endometriosis with a diagnostic laparoscopy, and for hysteroscopy to exclude pathological causes of intermenstrual bleeding
- Discuss risks of laparoscopic surgery (including increased risk from previous midline laparotomy of bowel injury)
- Advise to stop smoking

8 marks

Encounter 2
Laparoscopy
1 General anaesthesia to be administered. Patient placed in supine position with arms folded across chest, and legs in adjustable stirrups with knees bent, and hips in mild Trendelenberg position. Abdomen and then vulva and vagina to be prepped, followed by sterile draping. Bladder to be emptied with a urinary catheter.
2 Entry with Veress needle at Palmer's point (2 finger's breadth or 3 cm below left lower costal margin in mid-clavicular line) to minimise bowel injury at umbilical site from bowel adhesions from previous surgery. Insufflation of the abdomen to 15–20 mmHg pressure for port entry.
3 Insertion of other trocars under vision with 5 mm scope inserted at Palmer's point, including 10 mm scope at umbilical site if free of adhesions.
4 Pelvis to be visualised, with anteversion of the uterus via vaginal instrumentation. Any pathology to be photographed/documented, CO_2 gas to be emptied from abdomen and post sites sutured after completion of procedure.
(Alternative to Palmer's point entry is entry with the Hassan cannula – see discussion for description of technique)
Hysteroscopy: Vaginal examination to determine if uterus is anteverted or retroverted. Tenaculum or velsellum used to grasp the anterior lip of the

cervix prior to introduction of uterine sound. Cervix dilated to 6–7 Haegar, and hysteroscope introduced into uterine cavity with either CO_2 or saline used to dilate the cavity and provide adequate vision. A sharp curettage performed for endometrial sampling after cavity and ostia visualised at hysteroscopy.

3 marks

Encounter 3
• No change to history or examination. No complications from surgery. Laparoscopic wounds well healed.

Mrs KL has severe endometriosis. Her pain symptoms are likely to be due to the endometriosis. Best option for treatment is laparoscopic surgery with an experienced laparoscopic surgeon. She needs to be advised of:
• Need for bowel preparation (Golitely™ or Fleet™)
• Risk of damage to ureters, bladder, bowel, major blood vessels
• Involvement of colorectal surgeon, due to significant risk of damage to rectum
• Small risk of temporary colostomy if rectum damaged during excision of rectovaginal nodule
• Blood group and hold
• Need for admission to hospital at least overnight after surgery
• Consider combined oral contraceptive pill, medroxyprogesterone acetate 3-monthly depot injections, or Mirena IUD after surgery to minimise recurrence (patient refuses contraception)

2 marks

Encounter 4
1 Direct coupling:
  – current passes via direct contact from instrument to tissue
  – imperfect insulation of instrument, so electrical charge passes to contacted tissue
  – one metal instrument passes charge via another metal instrument to tissue
2 Thermal injury from heated instruments.
3 Capacitive coupling:
  – current passes indirectly from instrument to tissue
  – seen with mixed plastic/metal trocars, with lack of dissipation of current through abdominal wall
4 Sparks injuries
  – seen with prolonged application of current to already dessicated tissue; once resistance of tissue has reached a certain point, electrical current arcs unintentionally to adjacent moist tissue.

2 marks

Encounter 5

- Slight cramping pain in left iliac fossa. No vaginal bleeding. No bowel or urinary symptoms.
- Last menstrual period 6 weeks ago
- Abdomen soft
- Slight left adnexal tenderness on bimanual pelvic examination
- Urinary pregnancy test positive
- betaHCG = 2,400

Vaginal ultrasound
- Empty uterus. 2 cm left adnexal mass, with no FH visible. No free fluid in pelvis. Report: Likely left tubal ectopic pregnancy
- Patient does not want further laparoscopic surgery.
  "Are there any other options for treatment, doctor?"

Management
- Check FBE, urea + electrolytes + creatinine, liver function tests as baseline
- Check blood group (O negative), and administer 250 IU anti-D if needed
- Methotrexate 50mg/m^2 (body-surface area), or roughly 1mg/kg
- Check beta HCG on day 4 and day 7
- Recheck FBE, U+E, LFT on day 7
- If beta HCG drops by at least 15% from day 1 level on day 7 blood, can continue to monitor decline in betaHCG
- If fails to drop, or plateaus, or if pain/bleeding/rupture, needs laparoscopic salpingectomy/salpingostomy

5 marks
20 marks total

Discussion

The diagnosis in this case is simple, with endometriosis being the most likely cause of Mrs KL's symptoms. It is important that candidates avoid an umbilical entry in encounter 2 due to the risk posed by the previous midline laparotomy. Adhesions are likely after a ruptured appendix and subsequent surgery. An alternative to Palmer's point entry would be a Hassan cannula:
- Subumbilical incision, followed by elevation/incision of the fascia
- Visual confirmation of entry to the peritoneum
- Check for bowel in the vicinity of the incision
- If no bowel in the vicinity, 2 figure 8 sutures with 2–0 Vicryl placed and Hassan cannula inserted under direct vision.

All candidates should be familiar with and able to describe electrosurgical injuries at laparoscopic surgery, so as to be able to avoid them. They should also be able to identify the significant risk of rectal injury from surgical excision of the rectovaginal nodule described. Such surgery should usually be referred to a multi-disciplinary unit, if available, including experienced laparoscopic gynaecological surgeons, as well as a colorectal surgeon familiar with endometriosis surgery. It would be remiss not to warn of the risk of a temporary colostomy.

In the final encounter the candidate must ask for a history and examination to diagnose the tubal ectopic pregnancy. Endometriosis and adhesions from pelvic surgery are significant risk factors for ectopic pregnancies. Guidelines for administration of methotrexate vary at different institutions. As a rough guide, contraindications for methotrexate (and indication for surgery) include:

- patients with symptoms, or haemodynamically unstable
- high beta-HCG (>3,000 IU/l)
- tubal diameter >3 cm
- presence of fetal heart on ultrasound
- abnormal renal, liver or bone marrow function on pre-testing

The patient in this scenario has mild symptoms, but otherwise meets the criteria for methotrexate.

G7   Encounter 1
History
- Ms P, 26 years old
- G2P1 (previous NVD at term 2 years ago)
- Uncomplicated pregnancy up until now
- LMP 14 weeks and 5 days ago, no previous ultrasound
- PV bleeding started last night. Bright red blood, roughly a quarter of a cup in volume, now darkish
- Nausea and vomiting much more pronounced this pregnancy than in the last one
- Vomiting 2–3 times per day, despite using anti-emetics
- Blood group is rhesus positive
- Past medical history: appendicectomy at 15 y.o.; fractured femur at 18 y.o.
- Medications: Maxolon 10 mg QID
- Allergies: penicillin (rash)
- Non-smoker, no alcohol during pregnancy
- Family Hx: brother with type I insulin-dependent diabetes mellitus; mother with breast cancer aged 45 years old (alive and well)
- Social Hx: interior designer; husband is a newly qualified architect

3 marks

Encounter 2
- FBE
- U+E+creatinine
- LFTs
- Ultrasound scan
- Quantitative beta-HCG

2 marks

Encounter 3
The results of the ultrasound scan suggest a molar pregnancy. No fetal parts or gestational sac is seen.

The patient needs rehydration and a suction curettage.

2 marks

Encounter 4
Complete hydatidiform mole
- Lacks identifiable embryonic or fetal tissues. Shows diffuse hydatidiform swelling of the chorionic villi, and diffuse trophoblastic hyperplasia.
- Contains only paternal DNA, with an ovum lacking its own DNA fertilised by either a single haploid sperm (always 23X, 80%) that duplicates its chromosomes, or by two haploid sperm (23X + 23X, 10%; 23X + 23Y, 10%; never two 23Y sperm). Thus 90% have a karyotype of 46XX, and 10% 46XY.
- It has a 16% chance of progressing to an invasive mole, and 3% risk of developing into a choriocarcinoma if untreated.

Partial hydatidiform mole
- Has identifiable embryonic or fetal tissues
- Focal hydatidiform swelling, marked villous scalloping, and focal trophoblastic hyperplasia
- Prominent stromal trophoblastic inclusions
- Triploid (69 chromosomes), due to fertilisation of an ovum by 2 sperm
- Only a 0.5% chance of progressing to choriocarcinoma, less aggressive disease

6 marks

Encounter 5
- Weekly beta-HCGs until normal for 3 consecutive weeks, then monthly for 6 months
- Contraception during follow-up period to avoid confusion with a rising beta-HCG level
- Notification to a molar pregnancy register

2 marks

Encounter 6
- Complete history and examination
- Repeat beta-HCG
- FBE, U+E+creatinine, LFTs, TFTs
- CXR
- CT abdomen and pelvis
- CT or MRI head
- Measurement of cerebro-spinal fluid beat-HCG if any metastatic disease is present and the head CT is negative

3 marks

Encounter 7
- Single-agent chemotherapy: methotrexate with folic acid rescue
- Weekly beta-HCGs until normal for 3 weeks, then monthly until normal for 12 months
- Contraception for 12 consecutive months of normal beta-HCGs
- If fails to respond to methotrexate, treat with second-line combination chemotherapy (EMACO – etoposide, methotrexate, actinomycin-D, cyclophosphamide, vincristine)
- No damage to future fertility with either chemotherapy regime, and greater than 90% cure rate.

2 marks
20 marks total

Discussion
This OSCE is a relatively straightforward case of gestational trophoblastic disease with an invasive molar pregnancy requiring treatment with methotrexate. The incidence of complete molar pregnancies is estimated at about 1 per 1,000 pregnancies. The candidate is expected to display an understanding of the diagnosis and management of a molar pregnancy in this OSCE station.

G8 Q1
History
- 31-year-old G2P0 25/40 gestation (by early ultrasound)
- Past obstetric Hx: STOP at 8/40 when 18 years old
- Planned IVF pregnancy, pregnant on first cycle
- Infertility secondary to tubal damage (past Hx PID)
- Dichorionic diamniotic pregnancy on early ultrasound
- No problems with pregnancy up until now
- Antenatal investigations (on antenatal card):
  - Blood group AB POS, no antibodies
  - Haemoglobin 136 g/dl at 12/40, MCV 85, platelets 342
  - HepB/TPHA/HIV/MSU all negative
  - Rubella low immunity
  - 20/40 ultrasound: normal fetal anatomy (both fetuses); placentas not low-lying; anterior lower segment uterine fibroid 9 cm diameter, in a position to cause a risk of obstructed labour
- Small amount of fresh PV bleeding this morning, small clot on pad on arrival to delivery suite
- No associated pain; no rupture of membranes
- Fetal movements felt by patient
- Periods regular, 28 days apart and normal
- 2 episodes of PID secondary to chlamydia 10 years ago; tubal blockage discovered on investigation for infertility with laparoscopy 6/12 ago
- Last Pap smear 18 months ago normal (always normal)
- No medical problems

- No past surgery other than outlined above
- NKA medications: iron tablets
- Lives with husband (good relationship), non-smoker, non-drinker, no recreational drugs, works as a nail technician in a beauty parlour

4 marks, depending on completeness of history

Examination

- BP 120/60, PR 80, T 36.5 °C
- Abdominal Ex: symphyseal-fundal height = 28 cm, twin 1 transverse lie, twin 2 transverse lie, no fetal part in pelvis, fetal hearts both heard; uterus non-tender
- Speculum Ex: cervix 4 cm dilated with bulging membranes, slight bleeding from edge of cervix
- CTG of both twins (if asked for): normal for 25/40
- Ultrasound (available in labour ward if asked for): Both twins transverse lie, lower segment fibroid below twin 1

2 marks

Management

- Patient at risk of premature labour or premature rupture of membranes
- Need to transfer patient to a tertiary obstetric hospital as soon as possible
- Will need an escort (midwife or doctor)
- Maintain bed rest until transfer can be arranged
- Give betamethasone 11.4 mg IM (will need second dose in 24 hours)
- Give tocolysis (nifedipine orally) prior to transfer
- Obtain IV access for transfer

2 marks

Q2

The patient has had a cord prolapse. This is an obstetric emergency, and a life-threatening situation for the fetus.

N.B. Management occurring in the back of the ambulance

- Call for help – one of the ambulance team may be available to help, while the other drives
- Get the ambulance to call the hospital and get them to prepare theatre for an emergency classical caesarean section delivery. Will need to go straight from the ambulance to theatre on arrival at the hospital.
- Patient to position on all fours on the bed
- Place gloved hand into the vagina to elevate the presenting fetal part off the cord (prevent cord compression), and try to keep cord in the vagina (prevent cord spasm)
- Give O_2 by mask
- Obtain IV access (wide bore cannula) suitable for theatre on arrival

3 marks

Q3

- Patient wheeled into theatre as soon as arrives at the hospital

- Needs a general anaesthetic, with hand left holding cord and presenting fetal part right up until the patient is asleep (no time for a spinal/ epidural)
- In-dwelling catheter to be inserted and bladder emptied
- Patient to be prepped and draped after both fetal heart rates checked with doppler
- Can perform either an infra-umbilical vertical midline incision or a wide transverse Pfannensteil incision to skin
- Dissect down to rectus abdominis sheath; Cut sheath (vertically or horizontally, depending on skin incision)
- Enter peritoneal cavity
- Vertical incision to uterine body above the fibroid, taking care not to extend down to the bladder
- Delivery of both twins (by breech extraction)
- Delivery of placenta
- Closure of uterus in three layers of continuous sutures, ensuring adequate haemostasis
- Anticipate increased risk of post-partum haemorrhage due to fibroid
- Oppose edges of the serosal layer
- Close sheath with continuous layer
- Fat stitches (interrupted)
- Staples or subcutaneous continuous suture to skin

2 marks

Q4
History
- Twins left NICU a week ago, and are doing well
- Bleeding post-partum settled, now no bleeding
- Fully breastfeeding (no problems)
- Has not had sexual intercourse since delivery. Doesn't feel like it. Not using any contraception
- Has been crying a lot without any apparent reason. Feels not coping with the babies. Lack of energy and no interest in normal daily activities. Episodes of unprovoked anxiety since birth of the babies
- Not sleeping well, poor appetite
- Not feeling suicidal
- Not feeling any thoughts of wanting to harm the babies

1½ marks

Examination
- BP 120/80, PR 72
- Breasts – normal
- Abdomen – uterus just palpable above the symphysis pubis, C/S scar well healed
- Speculum/PV – bulky uterus with fibroid palpable, normal cervix (can take Pap smear)
- Babychecks of both babies normal

1½ marks

Management
- Candidate should recognise likely postnatal depression
- May need to use a validation technique such as the Edinburgh Postnatal Depression Scale (10 questions with answers scored between 0–3; if score 13 or more, likely to have postnatal depression)
- Needs review by a psychiatrist; if given an antidepressant, is still safe to continue breastfeeding; offer counselling + patient support groups

2 marks

- Needs rubella vaccine (low immunity)
- If due for Pap smear, repeat Pap smear
- Discussion about contraceptive options
- Needs to be informed that since she had a classical caesarean section she will need caesarean sections electively for any future pregnancies, due to risk of scar rupture

2 marks
20 marks total

Discussion
In this OSCE the candidate is expected to deal with a cord prolapse while in transit in an ambulance, and then describe their technique for a classical caesarean section. In the last encounter the patient presents with signs of postnatal depression, which she was at increased risk of given the dramatic nature of the delivery. The candidate is expected to diagnose and initiate management for the postnatal depression. All candidates for the specialist MRANZCOG exam should be familiar with the Edinburgh Postnatal Depression Scale.

MRANZCOG OSCE H

H1 Encounter 1
History
- 50-year-old woman
- Loses urine predominantly when coughing, laughing, sneezing, and with physical activity
- Needs to wear pads – using 4–5 pads per day
- Has needed to stop playing tennis due to the incontinence
- Frequency 8 times/day, nocturia 1 episode/night
- Occasional urgency and urge incontinence (1–2 episodes/week)
- No double voiding, no dysuria, no change in colour/smell of urine
- Limits water intake to reduce episodes of incontinence, 3 cups of coffee/day, no alcohol
- Bowel function normal – no constipation, eats adequate fibre; no incontinence of faeces or flatus
- Has not noticed a lump in the vagina

- No pain with sexual intercourse, does lose control of urine during sex, which has caused her to reduce sexual activity with her husband
- Periods increasingly irregular (regular up to 1 year ago), now only every 3–4 months
- Bleeding not heavy. Has a copper IUD in situ (inserted 5 years ago)
- Has been having hot flushes and night sweats lately, not bothering her much. Also has a dry vagina
- Last period 3 months ago, normal, always normal. Never had a mammogram
- No other past gynae history
- Para 4 – first was a forceps delivery, other 3 NVDs
- No past operations
- No family history of note
- Medical problems – swelling of the ankles, on Lasix 20 mg oral daily
- Lives with husband, primary school teacher, smokes 10 cigarettes per day, no alcohol/drugs
- Medications: Lasix 20 mg/day, NKA

Examination
- Normal general appearance
- PR 88, BP 130/70, T 37, RR 16, BMI 30, urinalysis normal
- Cardiorespiratory: crackles in lung bases, mild pitting oedema at ankles, otherwise normal
- Thyroid/breast normal
- Abdominal Ex: overweight, but normal
- Bimanual pelvic Ex: normal sized uterus, no adnexal masses, normal cervix on speculum Ex (can take smear) with strings visible
- Sims speculum Ex: grade 1 cystocele and uterine descent, no rectocele, stress incontinence demonstrated on coughing

Investigations/management
- Need MSU, urea and electrolytes, urodynamics, CXR, and Pap smear
- Encourage weight loss (? Refer to dietician, encourage exercise)
- Should stop smoking, reduce caffeine intake, and see if there is an alternative to Lasix treatment for her mild cardiac failure if possible (refer to physician)
- Copper IUD to be removed once menopause confirmed (1 year with no periods)
- Offer discussion regarding hormone therapy for menopausal Sx, including possible use of topical estrogen treatment to the vagina, such as Ovestin pessaries (patient happy to try estrogen pessaries, but not systemic hormone therapy)
- Check that baseline bone density scan, cholesterol/lipids have been checked
- Due for first mammogram (refer to Breastscreen)

8 marks

Encounter 2
- No change to history or Ex
- Pap smear, U+E, mammogram normal
- Options for management:
  - Pelvic floor exercises (patient has already tried them)
  - Surgical treatment – TVT procedure or Burch colposuspension
- Patient needs pre-operative work-up – review by physician, ECG, CXR
- Warn that will fix stress incontinence, but not urge (small risk of worsening existing mild urge incontinence)
- Counsel regarding risks of surgery – bleeding, infection, anaesthetic risks, damage to bladder/bowel, urinary retention, recurrent stress incontinence

4 marks

Encounter 3
- Patient generally feeling well
- PR 92, BP 135/75, T 37.2 °C
- Discharge foul-smelling and grey/watery; started 2 weeks ago; wet all the time, even at night
- No vaginal bleeding
- Abdominal Ex: normal
- Speculum Ex: granulation tissue at the vault, with fluid leaking from the granulation tissue
- Tampon test with indigo carmine – positive for urinary bladder fistula
- Cystogram – fistula between bladder and vagina
- Cystoscopy – urinary fistula to vaginal vault
- Management – involve urologist
  - Can try catheter and antibiotics for 2 weeks
  - If no spontaneous closure, need surgical dissection and repair in layers, with continuous bladder drainage for 10–12 days after repair, laxatives to reduce straining, and no intercourse or pessaries for 3 months; 80% cure rate.

4 marks

Encounter 4
- Itchy vulva, worse at night
- No bleeding, discharge, or ulceration/lumps
- No periods for 10 months, hot flushes reducing
- Has been very uncomfortable with sexual intercourse lately
- Urinary fistula completely healed, no stress incontinence and minimal urge incontinence
- On examination of vulva – atrophy of labia minora, thickened white plaques over labia and clitoris
- Biopsy confirms *lichen sclerosus*
- Management – topical steroid creams nightly for 4–6 weeks, then reducing to 2–3 times per week if symptoms controlled

- Needs vulvoscopy every 12 months due to increased risk of SCC vulva

4 marks

20 marks total

Discussion

This case requires the candidate to demonstrate the taking of a detailed urogynaecology history to arrive at the diagnosis. When a patient presents with urinary symptoms, other key features of the history are to ask about prolapse, bowel symptoms and sexual problems (often, but not always associated with urinary problems). The good candidate will demonstrate a consideration of the broader health issues for this woman, such as menopause, smoking, weight and lifestyle issues, as well as the medical problems, such as her mild cardiac failure.

Urinary fistulae are rare after surgery, but a specialist must understand the diagnosis and treatment of this potential complication of urogyaecological surgery. This is outlined in the answer to encounter 3.

Lichen sclerosus is the most common benign vulval condition to present to the gynaecologist. As such, specialist candidates are expected to be able to diagnose and treat this disorder.

H2 Q1

History

- Mrs Bryant, 24-year-old primigravida
- Singleton intrauterine pregnancy at 10/40 by early ultrasound
- Planned, spontaneous pregnancy
- Was on folate at time of conception
- Has been vomiting for the last week, unable to keep fluids down
- Feeling unwell with palpitations, agitation, and heat intolerance
- Not sleeping well lately
- Has had antenatal testing with her local doctor:
  - Blood group A POS, no antibodies; Hb 130, MCV 90; HepBsAg neg; TPHA neg; rubella immune; HIV neg; MSU no growth
- Periods regular 28 days apart, not heavy/painful
- No PHx gynaecological problems; Pap smears normal (last one 4/12 ago)
- No past medical or surgical Hx
- No family Hx of note
- NKA; Meds – folate
- Lives with husband, works as secretary, non-smoker, no alcohol/drug use

2½ marks

Examination

- Looks unwell and tired; visible tremor in hands
- Reduced skin turgor
- BMI 18; urinalysis ketones ++, nil else
- BP 100/60, PR 120 regular, RR 12, T 36.8 °C
- Thyroid Ex: palpable smooth goitre, with audible bruit on auscultation
- Cardio-respiratory Ex: normal

- Abdominal Ex: normal
- PV/speculum: 10/40 anteverted uterus, no adnexal masses, cervix appears normal

2½ marks

Management
- Patient is clearly dehydrated
- Admit, IV rehydration (4% in 1/5 normal saline)
- Add thiamine replacement (preferably intravenously) to prevent risk of Wernicke's encephalopathy (rare complication of severe hyperemesis gravidarum)
- Treatment of nausea: Pyridoxine orally 25 mg TDS, metoclopramide 10 mg IV TDS, ondansteron if does not respond to metoclopramide
- To try eating small regular, bland snacks, rather than attempt to eat big meals

2 marks

- Need to discuss Down syndrome screening (patient declines)

½ mark

- Patient has signs and symptoms suggestive of thyrotoxicosis
- Need thyroid function tests (free T4 and TSH levels), as well as thyroid auto-antibodies if hyperthyroidism confirmed

1½ marks

Q2
The tests show that Mrs Bryant has thyrotoxicosis (Grave's disease). She will require management in conjunction with an endocrinologist.

Radioactive iodine is contraindicated in pregnancy. Surgical treatment (subtotal thyroidectomy) is rarely required and best deferred until after pregnancy where indicated.
- Medical treatment the preferred option: PTU (propylthiouracil) 50 mg–150 mg daily, with dose titrated against thyroid function tests; Propranolol can be used to control heart rate
- Need to recheck thyroid function tests every month until stable and adjust dose of PTU to keep T4 levels at upper end of normal
- Can have a normal vaginal delivery

2½ marks

Risks to fetus
- Increased risk of IUGR (fetal biometry in third trimester) and premature labour
- Neonatal hypothyroidism and goitre secondary to PTU crossing placenta (need to check fetal TFTs after delivery), but effects usually short term
- Neonatal Graves' disease (10% risk) from auto-antibodies crossing placenta: tachycardia, LBW
- Breastfeeding acceptable as long as required PTU dose <150 mg/day

1½ marks

Q3
History
- 36/40 breech, normal growth on fetal biometry
- On 100 mg PTU daily with normal TFTs, feeling well
- Gestational diabetes screen negative at 28/40; 20/40 U/S normal fetus, placenta fundal
- Fetal movements normal

½ mark

Examination
- Well-looking, no tremor
- BP 110/60 PR 84
- Fundus = dates, breech presentation, fetal heart heard

½ mark

Counsel Mrs Bryant of the risks of a breech vaginal delivery (Term Breech Trial showed three-fold increased risk of adverse neonatal outcome with planned vaginal breech delivery compared with planned elective caesarean section).

1 mark

Options
1 Planned elective caesarean section at 38–39/40
2 External cephalic version – 66% chance of turning baby to cephalic presentation

PROMPT: "I like the idea of the baby being turned so I can have a vaginal delivery, but how is it done? Are there any risks?"
- Must exclude contraindications (e.g. placenta praevia, APH, PPROM, fetal anomalies, labour, multiple pregnancy)
- Relative contraindications: PHx LUSCS, oligohydramnios, IUGR
- Need to perform in centre with rapid access to C/S (< 1 in 1,000 risk of cord compression, CTG abnormalities requiring immediate delivery)
- Need normal CTG before, and CTG check after the ECV
- Tocolysis (nifedipine oral) preferable
- Anti-D if rhesus negative

2 marks

Q4
Diagnosis: inverted uterus

Management
- Call for help
- IV resuscitation
- Immediate attempt at digital replacement of the uterus into the pelvis
- If unsuccessful – consider further attempts at digital replacement in theatre with aid of tocolytic agents (GTN, halothane, salbutamol, terbutaline, etc)
- If fails, try O'Sullivan's hydrostatic method (4–5 L of warm saline instilled into vagina with hand occluding the introitus)

- If fails, need laparotomy

3 marks

20 marks total

Discussion

Hyperemesis gravidarum is a common symptom and condition in early pregnancy. Where the condition is severe enough to cause dehydration and require admission to hospital, rare causes should be excluded, such as hydatidiform molar pregnancy and thyrotoxicosis. In this case, an early ultrasound has excluded a molar pregnancy, but there are signs and symptoms suggestive of thyrotoxicosis.

Graves' disease is responsible for about 90% of cases of hyperthyroidism in pregnancy. The candidate is expected to display a knowledge of the diagnosis and management of the condition in the pregnant patient. There are potential fetal and neonatal consequences of both the condition and its treatment, as outlined in the model answer above.

The last two encounters require the candidate to manage a breech presentation at a gestation suitable for an external cephalic version, and then to manage an inverted uterus (an obstetric emergency).

H3 Encounter 1

History

- Miss P, 25 years old, nulliparous
- Regular periods, on the oral contraceptive pill
- Last Pap smear 6 months ago (normal; no past abnormal smears)
- Past Hx: tonsillectomy (7 years old); wisdom teeth extraction (19 years old)
- Family Hx
  - Mother – stage 3C serous papillary adenocarcinoma of ovary (44 years old). Treated with surgery, and now on her second cycle of chemotherapy.
  - Two maternal aunts with breast cancer (aged 43 years and 52 years at diagnosis)
  - Maternal grandmother died of cancer (? Ovarian possibly. "She had an abdomen full of fluid") at age 47
  - Miss P has 2 brothers, and a sister aged 14 years
  - No cancer on the paternal side of the family
- Ethnic background: Eastern European (Ashkenazi Jewish)
- University student, non-smoker, non-drinker, long-term boyfriend
- NKA medications (oral contraceptive pill)

5 marks

Encounter 2

There are several reasons why Miss P is at high risk of development of a malignancy:

1 She has one first-degree relative (her mother) with confirmed ovarian
   cancer.
   Most cases of ovarian cancer are sporadic. The lifetime risk of ovarian
   cancer in the general population is 1.4–1.8%. The risk for women with
   a single affected first-degree relative increases to 5–8%. With two or
   more affected relatives, the risk increases to 7–10%.
   However, approximately 5–10% of ovarian cancers are hereditary.
2 It is likely the patient's grandmother had ovarian cancer, suggesting
   a hereditary ovarian cancer syndrome.
3 Both her mother and her grandmother had their cancers at an early
   age (44 years and 47 years, respectively, well below the average age).
   This suggests a hereditary cancer, as hereditary ovarian cancer has
   a younger age of onset than sporadic cancer.
4 Two maternal aunts with breast cancer, again at an earlier age than
   average.

All of the above suggest a breast/ovarian cancer syndrome.
Miss P's family history of breast cancer in premenopausal women also
affects her risk of ovarian cancer (it approximately doubles it).

6 marks

Encounter 3
- BRCA1/BRCA2
- Lifetime risk of ovarian cancer with BRCA1 is 40%

2 marks

Encounter 4
Miss P needs referral to an hereditary/familial cancer clinic for counselling
regarding gene testing for BRCA1/2, and, if she wishes to proceed, for
genetic testing.

1 mark

Encounter 5
Miss P needs to be counselled together with her partner regarding the risks
of breast and ovarian cancers, including surgical options for prevention
(bilateral mastectomy and bilateral salpingo-oophorectomy).

The youngest case of breast cancer in the family was at 43 years of age.
Thus, Miss P is at greatest risk from the age of 33 years (10 years earlier than
the age of the earliest known case).

Options
- Surveillance and have a family
- Bilateral mastectomy and bilateral salpingo-oophorectomy

Surveillance
- Breast: 6-monthly mammograms (MRI may be more relevant in the
  not too distant future)

- Ovary: 6-monthly CA125 and pelvic examination and yearly pelvic ultrasound, but no proven benefit of screening for ovarian cancer
- There is no proven screening test for ovarian cancer (50% of stage 1 ovarian cancers do not have an elevated CA125)

Advised to start a family as soon as possible, followed by prophylactic bilateral salpingo-oophorectomy when family complete or by age 35 years.

If she doesn't want to get pregnant immediately, can consider the oral contraceptive pill as prophylactic treatment to prevent ovarian cancer, but there is some debate as to the usefulness of this measure in hereditary ovarian cancers (proven only for sporadic cancer cases).

6 marks
20 marks total

Discussion
This OSCE is largely a counselling station about BRCA gene mutations and the risk of familial ovarian cancer. The candidate is required to take a detailed family history, and deal sensitively with the uncovered BRCA1 gene mutation in a young woman.

H4 Encounter 1
History
- Mrs Rajendran, a 30-year-old Indian woman
- LMP 2 weeks ago. Menarche 14 years old; periods regular, 28 days apart, Bleeds have been increasingly heavy over the last 6 months, bleeding for 7–10 days, flooding and clots, uses 10 pads per day during period. Associated dysmenorrhoea for 3 days, but able to function normally during that time. No IMB/PCB. Has tried NSAIDs with GP, with no effect.
- Has been feeling tired and lethargic recently. Husband has commented that she is looking pale
- Sexually active for last 9 months (recently married), no dyspareunia, vaginal discharge, or past STDs
- Has never had a Pap smear
- Not using any contraception
- No past gynaecological history
- Nulliparous
- No past surgical or medical history, previously fit and well
- Family history: diabetes type 2 in father, mother had gestational diabetes
- Lives with husband (an accountant). Currently looking for work. Good relationship with husband, planning on starting a family soon. Non-smoker, no alcohol/drugs
- NKA; nil medications

Examination
- Pale conjunctivae, tired-looking

- PR 108, BP 90/55, T 37.2 ° C, RR 18
- BMI 20, urinalysis normal (pregnancy test negative if asked for)
- Thyroid, cardiovascular and breast Ex: all normal
- Abdominal Ex: normal
- Speculum Ex: Normal vulva, vagina, cervix, Pap smear can be taken
- Bimanual Ex: Anteverted, mobile, slightly bulky uterus, no adnexal masses

Investigations
- FBE: Hb 65, MCV 68, WCC 9.0, platelets 297
- Iron studies: Very low ferritin, increased total iron binding capacity
- Hb electrophoresis normal
- U+E+creatinine, TFTs, LFTs all normal
- APTT + INR normal
- Pap smear normal
- Pelvic ultrasound: Bulky anteverted uterus with a 4 cm pedunculated submucosal fibroid attached to the fundus and filling the uterine cavity. A 3 cm subserosal fibroid attached to the posterior surface of the uterus. Both ovaries normal in size and appearance

Management
Admit, as needs a blood transfusion of 2–3 units of packed cells
- Commence oral iron tablets and vitamin C tablets
- Need to plan for a hysteroscopic resection of submucosal fibroid, once haemodynamically stable
  - (Counsel re risks of general anaesthetic, incomplete resection and recurrence, perforation of uterus and damage to internal organs, water intoxication/electrolyte imbalances, bleeding, infection, scarring)

7 marks

Encounter 2
- Amenorrhoeic since surgery. No hot flushes. No acne, hirsutism, visual changes, galactorrhoea
- Otherwise well. Energy levels much improved
- Wants to try for a baby soon

Investigations
- Rubella low immune
- FSH, LH, Estradiol all within normal limits for premenopausal woman
- Ultrasound: Bulky Av uterus with subserosal fibroid previously noted
- Contrast hysterosonography, or hysterosalpingogram – shows moderate amount of scarring/synechiae consistent with Asherman's syndrome

Management
- Explain condition, a result of her surgery. Need for operation to correct, and risk of placenta accreta if ever gets pregnant
- Hysteroscopic resection of synechiae by experienced surgeon (may require laparoscopy to reduce risk of perforation) using hysteroscopic scissors (most operators avoid diathermy). Antibiotics to be given

perioperatively (amoxicillin and metronidazole), and use of Premarin 5 mg/day for 1 month post-operatively and 10 mg/day Provera for the last 10 days of the month to induce a withdrawal bleed (now standard post-operative management instead of an IUD)

- Good chances of pregnancy after operation, but risk of placenta accreta
- Needs rubella vaccination (must be pregnancy-free for 3 months after)
- If she gets pregnant, will need glucose tolerance test (family Hx of diabetes)

6 marks

Encounter 3

- Placenta accreta, therefore high likelihood of requiring a caesarian hysterectomy
- Patient will need to be consented for this possibility, as well as a general anaesthetic and a midline laparotomy
- Experienced surgeon, possibly a gynae-oncologist to be present or on standby in case of need for a caesarean hysterectomy
- 4–6 units of blood to be cross-matched
- Anaesthetic review/consultation, 2 experienced anaesthetists in OT, at least 2 large bore lines in situ – blood in theatre

2 marks

Encounter 4

- Patient feeling unwell
- Clear fluid 250 mLs drained from midline laparotomy wound
- Diffuse abdominal pain and discomfort
- Urine output >30 mLs/hour
- Minimal blood loss from vagina
- Post-operative Hb 110 yesterday
- Baby is well, bottlefeeding
- Mild temperature 37.8 °C, PR 110, BP 90/60
- Diffuse peritonism and rebound tenderness, reduced bowel sounds

Investigation

- FBE Hb 108, WCC 15.0, platelets 320
- U+E+creatinine: normal
- If fluid leaking from wound collected, creatinine levels elevated
- IVP – Left ureter transected just below the pelvic brim. Right ureter intact.

Management

- Call in urologist. Will need open repair with Boari bladder flap procedure

5 marks
20 marks total

Discussion

This case requires the candidates to take a history from a woman with menorrhagia, and then move through a series of encounters including obstetric and post-operative scenarios. The candidates are expected to demonstrate an ability to diagnose and manage Asherman's syndrome in encounter 2. This is outlined in the model answer above. The placenta accreta in encounter 3 should already have been anticipated by the fact that the patient has Asherman's syndrome and is pregnant. The candidates should not forget simple pre-pregnancy tests such as rubella (here the patient required rubella vaccination), and should use information given in the initial history in later encounters (such as the family history of gestational diabetes in the initial history for encounter 1, which becomes relevant in deciding on obstetric management).

Ureteric injuries during obstetric and gynaecologic surgery can be diagnosed at the time of surgery, but often have a delay in diagnosis. The earlier they are recognised, the better the prospects for repair. The best test for diagnosis is an intravenous pyelogram or a CT scan with contrast.

Surgical repair depends on the level of the injury:

- Lower third of ureter – reimplantation of ureter into bladder (+/- Psoas hitch procedure)
- Middle third – Boari flap
- Upper third – end to end anastomosis of ureter (uretero-ureterostomy) with stent insertion.

While obstetricians and gynaecologists would not be expected to know how to perform these operations, which are performed by urologists, it is reasonable to expect examination candidates for the specialty exams to know what methods of repair are available, as urinary tract injuries are relatively common.

H5 Q1

History

- 25-year-old nulliparous
- Type 1 DM: diagnosed 10 years ago, using Mixtard 30/70 20 units mane + 24 units in the evening. No lipodystrophy or tachyphylaxis from insulin use
- Checks BSLs 1–2 times/day, varying testing time. BSLs 8–12 recently
- Last HbA1C 10% 3/12 ago. Has endocrinologist, but sees her infrequently
- Had 1 episode of ketoacidosis 2 years ago
- Gets 2–3 UTIs every year
- No long-term complications: last microalbuminuria checked 3/12 ago (negative); last eye check 3 years ago (normal)
- Married 2 years ago, and would like to try for a baby soon
- Rubella not checked. No pre-pregnancy investigations yet
- Not on folate/multivitamins
- Gynae Hx:

- Menarche at 13 y.o.; LMP 7/7 ago; periods regular every 28 days lasting 3 days, not heavy or painful, no intermenstrual or post-coital bleeding; no discharge or STDs; last Pap smear 6/12 ago normal, but had CIN2 treated 4 years ago with cone biopsy; using condoms for contraception
- No past medical/psychiatric Hx
- Past surgical Hx: cone biopsy 4 years ago
- No family Hx of note
- Lives with husband, good relationship, works at a call centre, smokes 10 cigarettes per day, drinks alcohol occasionally, no recreational drugs
- NKA. Meds – Mixtard 30/70 as above

4 marks

Examination
- Normal general appearance
- BP 120/70, PR 72, T 36.8 °C, RR 12
- Urinalysis negative; BMI = 20
- Thyroid, breast, cardiorespiratory, neurological Ex: all normal
- Abdominal Ex: normal
- PV/speculum Ex: normal

1 mark

Investigations/management
- Stop smoking – risks to maternal health (ischaemic heart disease, peripheral vascular disease, lung disease, cancer) and fetal health (IUGR/FDIU/SIDS)
- No safe level of alcohol consumption in pregnancy – stop during pregnancy, and while trying to conceive. Can also have effects on blood sugar levels
- Needs to start folate/multivitamins (to reduce risk of neural tube defects)
- Needs rubella serology check
- Recurrent UTIs: will need MSU at least once/trimester, and prompt treatment of infections. Consider prophylactic antibiotics (nitrofurantoin 100 mg nocte)
- Past Hx of cone biopsy: increases risk of cervical incompetence; suggest cervical tracking with ultrasound every 2/52 from 14/40 till 24/40

½ mark for each point (3 marks maximum)

Type I diabetes
Multidisciplinary management (involve endocrinologist, diabetes educator, dietician, tertiary obstetrics unit).

Pre-pregnancy
- Improve BSLs to reduce risk of fetal congenital defects (fasting < 6 mmol/L, post-prandial < 7 mmol/L, HbA1C < 8%)
- Increase frequency of BSL testing
- Change to Actrapid TDS and Protaphane nocte, either before or early in pregnancy

- Needs eye check (ophthalmologist) + renal function assessment (24-hour urine protein and creatinine clearance, urea and electrolytes)

Antenatal
- Maternal
  - Need more frequent monitoring of BSLs (risk of hypoglycaemic episodes in T1, and of diabetic ketoacidosis in T2–3 due to changing insulin requirements
  - If abnormal renal function or retinopathy, risk of progression in pregnancy
  - Increased infections (UTI, thrush, endometritis and mastitis post-partum)
  - Increased polyhydramnios, macrosomia (traumatic delivery, shoulder dystocia, instrumental and C/S delivery, PPH), pre-eclampsia (need more frequent visits with BP/urine dipstick monitoring)
- Fetal
  - Increased congenital malformations (reduce with tight BSL control): need teriary level ultrasound at 20/40 and again at 22/40 for better cardiac views
  - Increased risk of preterm birth, miscarriage, IUGR, FDIU, macrosomia, polyhydramnios: need 4/52ly fetal biometry from 28/40, CTGs twice/week from 32/40, and may recommend C/S if U/S shows fetal weight > 4 kg
  - Neonatal risks: respiratory distress syndrome, hypoglycaemia, hypocalcemia, jaundice/polycythaemia (admit to NICU post-delivery)

Delivery
- Can go to term if no complications
- Insulin/dextrose infusion in labour; back to pre-pregnancy insulin levels after birth

4 marks

Q2
History
- 19/40 by early ultrasound; fetal movements felt occasionally; feels well
- Last HbA1C 7%; has worked hard to improve control of BSLs
- Renal/eye checks normal
- On Actrapid 12 units TDS and protaphane 10 units nocte (BSLs 6–8 mmol/L)
- Feels slight pressure in vagina, no discharge
- Patient very worried about risk to pregnancy

Examination
- BP 110/70; urinalysis trace protein

- Fundal height appropriate for dates. Fetal heart heard with doppler
- Sterile speculum Ex: cervix 3 cm dilated with slight bulge of membranes visible

1 mark

Management
- Explain likely cervical incompetence due to past Hx of cone biopsy
- Admit patient; bed rest (head slightly down)
- No intercourse or vaginal examinations
- Needs insertion of cervical suture (McDonald's or Shirodkar): risk of bleeding, infection, PPROM

2 marks

Q3
- Patient to be consented, given a general anaesthetic, placed in lithotomy, prepped and draped, and the bladder emptied
- A 2-PDS suture on a large curved needle used to form a purse-string suture after gently pushing the bulging membranes back to the level of the internal os. The purse-string to be started from the superior aspect of the cervix, at the level of the internal os, with the knot to be tied superiorly to the cervix
- Consider nifedipine 20 mg TDS for 2 days as tocolysis, and oral antibiotics. Maintain bed rest for 2–3 days post procedure

2 marks

Q4
History
- Dysuria and urinary frequency for last 2 days
- Started leaking watery fluid 3 hours ago; initial gush, now steady loss
- Some cramping abdominal pains; no PV bleeding
- Fetal movements present. No other changes

Examination
- BP 130/70, PR 100, T 38 °C, RR 20
- BSL 12 mmol/L
- Urinalysis leucocytes +++, red blood cells +++
- Abdomen – mild suprapubic tenderness, fetal heart +ve
- Sterile speculum – amniotic liquor leaking from internal os

1 mark

Management
- Likely PPROM post-UTI
- Admit patient
- Remove cervical suture (risk of infection)
- IV antibiotics for UTI after sending off an MSU for culture
- Increase insulin for BSL control
- Consider betamethasone for fetal lung maturation (but may worsen BSLs)

- Ultrasound for biometry, biophysical profile, AFI
- Counsel patient about the risk of preterm delivery, and ask neonatologist to discuss prognosis for the baby with the mother
- Other risks from low liquor volume: pulmonary hypoplasia, limb contractures, Potter's facies

2 marks
20 marks total

Discussion

This OSCE requires the candidate to manage two potential problems in pregnancy: type I diabetes and cervical incompetence.

The unfortunate patient presented in this scenario develops cervical incompetence, which the candidate is required to successfully treat with a cervical suture. Then the patient develops a urinary tract infection, causing premature rupture of the membranes. There is a high risk of premature delivery of the fetus owing to both the PPROM and the urinary tract infection, both of which can precipitate preterm labour. Therefore, careful counselling to the patient about the risk of this to the baby is paramount.

H6 Encounter 1

History

- Mrs P, 32 years old
- Regular menstrual cycle with no intermenstrual or post-coital bleeding
- G2P1 (PHx NVD at term 2 years ago; son, alive and well)
- Recent thrush, self-treated with vaginal anti-fungal
- No history of genital warts or herpes
- Past Hx: tonsillectomy (aged 4); appendicectomy (aged 21); knee reconstruction (aged 28)
- No regular medications; no known allergies
- Non-smoker
- Family Hx: maternal aunt died of cervical cancer aged 47
- Lives with husband and child; competitive netball player (state level)

3 marks

Encounter 2

- Colposcopic examination of the cervix, using 5% acetic acid to identify dysplastic areas; cervical biopsy to be taken from any aceto-white stained areas
- Repeat Pap smear
- High vaginal swab
- (Optional: high-risk HPV DNA test – may be useful in triaging possible high-grade lesion)

EXAMINER: "Transformation zone in view; dense aceto-white staining on anterior and posterior lips of the cervix; upper extent of the lesion visible with manipulation of the cervix."

4 marks

Encounter 3

Results show high-grade changes in both squamous and glandular cells in the transformation zone of the cervix (pre-cancerous changes to the cells of the cervix – not actual cancer).

These changes are caused by the human papilloma virus. This is not a single virus but a large family of viruses (to date >200 identified). At least 30 types of HPV infect the human genital tract. Of these, 18 are recognised as being oncogenic (causing abnormally excessive growth of the cells of the cervix), and have been associated with the eventual occurrence of cervical cancer (16, 18, 26, 31, 33, 35, 39, 45, 51, 52, 53, 56, 58, 59, 66, 68, 73, and 82).

HPV 16, 18, 31, and 45 account for 80% of cervical cancers.

The high-risk HPV DNA test detects 13 of the high-risk virus sub-types (16, 18, 31, 33, 35, 39, 45, 51, 52, 56, 58, 59, 68). These oncogenic types are the cause of the high-grade lesions, both squamous and glandular.

While high-grade lesions can resolve spontaneously, the viral infection can also persist and lead to the development of cervical carcinoma. Hence all high-grade lesions require treatment.

The appropriate treatment for Mrs P is a cold-knife cone biopsy due to the presence of adenocarcinoma in situ (ACIS).

ACIS occurs in the glandular cells of the endocervix higher up the cervical canal. It represents a field change to the glandular epithelium of the uterus, and is often multi-focal. Women are advised to complete their family relatively promptly, and consider a hysterectomy once their family is complete.

3 marks

Encounter 4

- Infection
- Bleeding (<10% may have bleeding requiring vaginal packing or a blood transfusion. **Very** rarely need hysterectomy for uncontrolled bleeding)
- Cervical incompetence
- Cervical stenosis
- Further treatment (incompletely resected lesion/recurrent lesion)

3 marks

Encounter 5

History
- No chills/fevers/rigors
- History of bleeding onset and severity given in question

Examination
- BP 100/60, PR 106, Temp 37.1 °C
- Speculum Ex: obvious bleeding point on cervix

Management
- IV access and fluid replacement
- Bloods for FBE, group and hold, cross-match blood, coagulation profile (no need for blood cultures, as temp <38 °C)
- Commence IV antibiotics
- Apply pressure at the bleeding point on cervix to stop bleeding
- Insert vaginal pack
- Insert urinary catheter

2 marks

Encounter 6
- Continue resuscitation (fluids, blood, blood products if coagulopathy)
- Arrange theatre
- Examine in lithotomy, with adequate light and suction

Options
- Diathermy to cervix (unlikely to work)
- Suture to cervix

If continues to bleed.
- Correct coagulopathy
- Continue fluid resuscitation
- Hysterectomy OR (if available) embolisation

5 marks
20 marks total

Discussion
The candidate is expected to understand the aetiology and management of both squamous and glandular cervical dysplasia. This is a straightforward OSCE dealing with a common and important clinical problem, and candidates at specialist level would be expected to perform well at this station.

H7 **Encounter 1**
History
- 28 years old
- Menarche 13 years
- Regular periods until 5 years ago. Periods were every 28–30 days, lasting 5 days with no problems. Periods then became irregular, often months apart and now no period for the past 2 years
- For the past 5 years has had hot flushes and particularly night sweats that are preventing sleep and causing a lot of tiredness. Symptoms are becoming worse. Also more irritable, gets upset easily
- Married 6 months ago. Was using condoms until 6 months ago but not now as wants to have a child. Pain with intercourse due to vaginal dryness. Pap smear normal 6 months ago
- No past history – medical or surgical
- Mother has type II diabetes and went through menopause at 44 years, father has had a heart attack at age 55

- No allergies, no medications, non-smoker, occasional alcohol

4 marks

Examination
- BP 120/70, PR 80, T 37
- Normal general appearance
- Cardiovascular/respiratory/breast/thyroid Ex: normal
- Abdominal Ex: NAD
- Pelvic Ex: normal

2 marks

Investigations
- FSH and LH (check on two separate occasions), prolactin, TSH

2 marks

Encounter 2
It is expected that the candidate will interpret the results correctly, showing that the patient has premature ovarian failure (POF).

The candidate needs to discuss the results with empathy, understanding that the diagnosis will be devastating to a young woman.

2 marks

Further investigations necessary
- Karyotype, once hormonal profile known
- Bone density, once hormonal profile known
- Vitamin D, once bone density known

3 marks

Encounter 3
The candidate is also expected to interpret the bone density showing moderate osteopaenia and that the vitamin is low in the presence of a low bone density and requires treatment with 1 tablet of Ostelin or Osteovit and that the vitamin D needs repeating to make sure replacement is adequate.

2 marks

The candidate is expected to discuss options for treatment of menopausal symptoms. The option is HT, given that the patient wants to become pregnant. The ideal option is a sequential regimen of treatment so that if spontaneous pregnancy occurs by chance it can be suspected due to the lack of a withdrawal bleed. The HT will improve the symptoms and prevent further bone loss in combination with adequate vitamin D replacement. The issue of the risks of HT in the older menopausal woman is not relevant to this patient given the diagnosis of POF.

The patient is begun on a sequential dose of HT and the side effects of breast tenderness and withdrawal bleed are discussed, as well as the positive treatment benefits of treatment of symptoms, including vaginal dryness and bone protection.

3 marks

Options for future pregnancy need to be discussed. Once again, this needs to be discussed in an empathetic manner, discussing that the chance of spontaneous pregnancy is low and that the best chance of pregnancy will be with the use of donor eggs.

2 marks
20 marks total

Discussion
This is a counselling station and it is expected that the candidate will discuss the patient's concerns in plain language and treat the patient with empathy. The expectation is that the candidate will take an adequate history such that POF is suspected and that the investigations are appropriate for diagnosing the problem and excluding other causes for the history. Given the patient has been menopausal for the past 2 years it is expected that the candidate will discuss the use of hormone therapy (HT) as the patient has menopausal symptoms, and, in addition, will discuss bone protection. As the patient wants to have a child the probability of spontaneous pregnancy will need to be discussed as well as the treatment option of donor eggs. Marks will not be awarded for investigations that are not appropriate.

H8   Q1
History
- 29-year-old nulliparous woman
- Married 2 years ago. She and her husband now wish to start their family
- SLE diagnosed 5 years ago after the onset of a photosensitive skin rash and joint pains. Sees a rheumatologist for management of the condition
- When disease flares she gets joint pains, especially in her hands, and a skin rash on her face. Last flare-up was 9 months ago. She is unaware of her test results ("I leave that up to my rheumatologist")
- No known effects on kidneys, heart, or platelets. No history of DVT/PE
- Currently treated with prednisolone 10 mg oral daily and Plaquenil 400 mg oral daily; has had methotrexate and cyclophosphamide to treat flares in the past (last episode 9 months ago)
- Periods regular and not heavy or painful. Pap smear 6/12 ago, normal. Using condoms for contraception
- No other medical problems. No past surgical history
- No family history of note
- Non-smoker, non-drinker; drug and alcohol counsellor; lives with husband in supportive relationship
- NKA. Medications – prednisolone, Plaquenil

(If the candidate starts asking about an examination, move them on with: "Her examination is normal. Please advise her on your management.")

4 marks

Investigations/management

Pregnancy should only be contemplated with SLE when stable (i.e. no recent flare-ups of disease). This patient appears to be stable.

While flare-ups of SLE can occur during pregnancy and post-partum, there appears to be no increased risk compared with non-pregnant state.

Her SLE should not affect her fertility, unless she has severe renal disease.

2 marks

Prednisolone is safe for pregnancy. Should not use methotrexate or cyclophosphamide in pregnancy (teratogenic). Plaquenil is probably safe in pregnancy, but may try to stop it in consultation with rheumatologist (may not be possible).

1 mark

Before it is possible to advise the patient about the safety of pregnancy, more information and investigation results need to be sought (can either request recent results from rheumatologist, or perform investigations):

- Full blood examination (assess for thrombocytopaenia, anaemia)
- Glucose tolerance test (check for diabetes due to long-term prednisolone use)
- Urea and electrolytes
- 24-hour urine protein; 24-hour urine creatinine clearance (assess renal function)
- Anti-nuclear antigen titre
- C3/C4 titres (if low, may be risk of a flare)
- Anti-dsDNA
- Anti-Ro/La antibody titres (if positive, risk of neonatal lupus in fetus)
- Anti-phospholipid antibodies/anticardiolipin antibodies (if positive, risk of DVT/PE in mother, and miscarriage/IUGR/FDIU in fetus)

3 marks (½ mark for each to maximum 3 marks)

Q2

The candidate is expected to counsel the patient about the risks of SLE and pregnancy in general, as well as specifically with the results of the investigations provided.

General risks of SLE

- Maternal – SLE flares; pre-eclampsia; hypertension of pregnancy
- Fetal – increased risk of miscarriage, IUGR, prematurity, perinatal mortality; neonatal lupus rare

1 mark

Worst risks to mother are with renal impairment from SLE, but Mrs Turnbull has normal renal function.

- Anti-Ro antibodies: 1% risk of neonatal lupus in fetus, characterised by:
  - haematological abnormalities (thrombocytopaenia, reduced WCC, anaemia)
  - complete heart block

- neonatal skin lesions on face/scalp (will resolve spontaneously)
- Caused by antibodies crossing the placenta to the fetus
- Need frequent assessment of fetal heart rate, and tertiary level fetal heart ultrasound assessment

1½ marks

Anticardiolipin antibodies:
- Risk of DVT/PE in mother
- Risk of miscarriage/fetal loss/IUGR increased over normal with SLE
- Need aspirin 100 mg daily, plus LMW heparin throughout pregnancy to reduce fetal effects
- Will need third trimester fetal growth scans and fetal monitoring (CTGs)

1½ marks

As with any woman contemplating pregnancy, need to check rubella serology, and start folate supplementation.

½ mark

Will need frequent visits during pregnancy (once per 1–2 weeks) with regular FBE, renal function tests (blood and 24-hr urine protein).

Patient will need to be managed in a tertiary hospital, as high-risk pregnancy.

Do not allow to go post-term. Will need hydrocortisone IV cover for delivery (as has had long-term prednisolone treatment).

1½ marks

Q3
History
- Pregnancy has progressed well. No flares-ups, no renal manifestations
- Mother and baby have progressed well
- All pregnancy investigations have been normal, including 20/40 ultrasound and glucose tolerance test
- Fetal movements reduced over last 2 days
- On aspirin and Clexane

Examination
- BP 120/80, PR 92, Looking well
- Abdominal Ex: fundus = dates; fetal heart rate 55–60 bpm with doppler, cephalic presentation, longitudinal lie
- PV Ex: Cervix long, closed and posterior

1 mark

Management
- Fetus likely has complete heart block secondary to neonatal lupus
- Need to alert the paediatric cardiology team
- Will need prompt delivery by caesarean section, once neonatologists/paediatric cardiologists prepared
- Mother will need IV hydrocortisone cover for delivery
- Will need to be aware of increased risk of operative bleeding associated with Clexane/aspirin. Have protamine-S on hand as well as prostaglandin F2 alpha

- After delivery, fetus will need stabilisation in NICU, assessment of haematological effects of neonatal lupus, and consideration of a permanent pacemaker to prevent/treat heart failure

3 marks
20 marks total

Discussion

Systemic lupus erythematosus, or SLE, is a multisystem auto-immune disorder. It has a prevalence of up to 0.1%, and is 10 times more prevalent in women than in men.

Diagnosis of SLE is based on the Americal Rhematology Association criteria (if any 4 or more of 11 criteria are met):

1 Malar rash
2 Discoid rash
3 Photosensitivity
4 Oral ulcers
5 Arthritis
6 Serositis
7 Renal disease: >0.5 f/d proteinuria, or >3+ dipstick proteinuria, or cellular casts
8 Neurologic disease: seizures, or psychosis (without other cause)
9 Hematologic disorders:
    a Hemolytic anemia, or
    b Leukopenia <400/uL, or
    c Thrombocytopenia <100,000/uL
10 Immunologic abnormalities:
    a Positive LE cell prep, or
    b Antibody to native DNA, or
    c Antibody to Sm, or
    d False-positive serologic syphilis test
11 Positive ANA test

Source: Tan EM, Cohen ES, Fries JF et al 1982 The 1982 revised criteria for the classification of systemic lupus erythematosus. Arthritis and Rheumatism 25(11):1271–1277

Since the disease often affects women in the reproductive age, when it is more readily diagnosed and more effectively treated, it is not uncommon for patients to wish to present desiring a pregnancy. A knowledge of the effects of SLE on both the mother and the fetus during pregnancy are assessed in this OSCE.

The last encounter requires the candidate to recognise complete heart block due to neonatal lupus, and to display a knowledge of appropriate management.

Index